DI014252

The Organic Nanny's Guide
to Raising Healthy Kids

The Organic Nanny's

GUIDE TO RAISING

Healthy Kids

How to Create a Natural Diet and Lifestyle for Your Child

BARBARA RODRIGUEZ
with Eve Adamson

Da Capo
LIFE
LONG

A Member of the Perseus Books Group

Copyright © 2012 by Barbara Rodriguez

All rights reserved. No part of this publication may be reproduced, stored in a retrieval system, or transmitted, in any form or by any means, electronic, mechanical, photocopying, recording, or otherwise, without the prior written permission of the publisher. Printed in the United States of America. For information, address Da Capo Press, 44 Farnsworth Street, 3rd Floor, Boston, MA 02210.

Designed by Brent Wilcox
Set in 11.25 point Kepler Std-Light by the Perseus Books Group

Library of Congress Cataloging-in-Publication Data
Rodriguez, Barbara.
   The organic nanny's guide to raising healthy kids : how to create a natural diet and lifestyle for your child / Barbara Rodriguez with Eve Adamson.
      p.   cm.
   Includes index.
   ISBN 978-0-7382-1489-4 (pbk.)—ISBN 978-0-7382-1530-3 (e-book)
   1. Children—Nutrition.   2. Natural foods.   3. Food habits.   4. Parenting.   I. Adamson, Eve.   II. Title.
   RJ206.R664 2012
   618.92—dc23

                                                                                    2011042717

First Da Capo Press edition 2012

Published by Da Capo Press
A Member of the Perseus Books Group
www.dacapopress.com

Note: The information in this book is true and complete to the best of our knowledge. This book is intended only as an informative guide for those wishing to know more about health issues. In no way is this book intended to replace, countermand, or conflict with the advice given to you by your own physician. The ultimate decision concerning care should be made between you and your doctor. We strongly recommend you follow his or her advice. Information in this book is general and is offered with no guarantees on the part of the authors or Da Capo Press. The authors and publisher disclaim all liability in connection with the use of this book. This book includes many stories about my clients and their children. In order to protect the identities and privacy of those children as well as their parents, all names and other identifying details have been changed, and in some cases, details from several different clients have been combined into one, or inspired by, but not directly based on, real events and people. Barbara Rodriguez is an experienced nanny, but not a medical professional. No information in this book is meant to replace the advice of a personal physician or other health care professional. Before making any drastic changes in your child's life, please consult your child's doctor. Barbara Rodriguez, Eve Adamson, and the publisher assume no responsibility for harm incurred based on any information or interpretation of information in this book.

Da Capo Press books are available at special discounts for bulk purchases in the U.S. by corporations, institutions, and other organizations. For more information, please contact the Special Markets Department at the Perseus Books Group, 2300 Chestnut Street, Suite 200, Philadelphia, PA, 19103, or call (800) 810-4145, ext. 5000, or e-mail special.markets@perseusbooks.com.

10 9 8 7 6 5 4 3 2 1

This book is dedicated to my angels in heaven—
my parents, and of course, my Tata. You are missed.

Also to my soul sister Annie, and to all the amazing children,
mamas, and nannies—may you carry the organic message.

Contents

Acknowledgments   ix

INTRODUCTION
A Legacy of Love   1

CHAPTER ONE
Food, L.O.V.E., and Healing   11

CHAPTER TWO
Step 1: Eliminate the Worst Offenders
from Your Child's Diet   27

CHAPTER THREE
Step 2: Sugar Freedom   51

CHAPTER FOUR
Step 3: Phase Out White Flour,
Embrace Whole Grains   65

CHAPTER FIVE
Step 4: Ditch Dairy and Change Your Life   75

CHAPTER SIX
Step 5: Eat More Veggies, Less Meat,
and with L.O.V.E.   85

CHAPTER SEVEN
Putting the Pieces Together   109

CHAPTER EIGHT

Detoxing Your Home   133

CHAPTER NINE

Phenomenal Mama Makeover   147

CHAPTER TEN

Natural Remedies from the Botanica   173

CHAPTER ELEVEN

An Attitude of Gratitude   193

CHAPTER TWELVE

Listen from the Heart   209

Appendix One: Organic Nanny Kid-Friendly Recipes   225

Appendix Two: Organic Nanny Resources   247

Index   251

Acknowledgments

I am so incredibly grateful to the extraordinary people who helped make my dream come true.

First, my heartfelt thanks go to my incredible agent, Sarah Jane Freymann, who believed in me from the start and guided me with her knowledge and deep intuitive wisdom.

I am deeply thankful to Eve Adamson for bringing her talent to this project. I knew from our first conversation that she was a sister in my organic revolution and understood my philosophies. I am grateful for her friendship and her hard work.

Thank you to Jamie Babbitt, a wonderful writer, singer, and great friend.

I am also grateful to my editor, Katie McHugh, for her ongoing support.

I appreciate all my beautiful little clients that have touched my heart and made me smile. I am grateful to have shared in their lives. And to all my furry clients, you still live in my heart.

I want to acknowledge all the beautiful people in my life who have inspired and held me together: Susan and Sierra, Anne Dial, and Tommy, Paula Murphy, and Chix Nana, Melanie Banks, LeAna M., Emily L., Cynthia F., and Roxie, Chrissy and Maria, Anne Wilde and her bro Scottie, Sheila, and Angelique, Frank, Nene, Buddy Allen, Taresa, and Brody, Barbara Muncy, Karen Garcia, my teachers Gabrielle M., Natalia Rose, Louise L. Hay, Mama Maria Rodriguez.

And to my mentors: Julia L. for the wisdom and Kenny for the Husband; Bethenny F., you inspired the dream; Nicole K., thank you for the words "Beautiful Barbara"; Eva Peron; and John Lennon and the summer of L.O.V.E.

And finally, to Chris, Andre, and my fabulously organic Nicki—I love you!

A Legacy of Love

Our children are all on a journey and constantly blooming.
—The Organic Nanny

*M*y name is Barbara Rodriguez, and I am the Organic Nanny. For more than twenty years, I have taken care of children as a profession. I have worked with a wide range of culturally diverse children ranging in age from eleven months to sixteen years old, and I've forged unique and lasting relationships with them all. I work within a rich and privileged world—many of the children I work with have celebrity parents—but I believe all children can benefit from the changes I help my clients realize. Those changes are all, at their essence, organic, and by that I mean natural, life-giving, and in harmony with the spirit and essence of the individual child. Organic food, organic relationships, and an organic connection with the Earth can revitalize and optimize every child's life.

In my work as a nanny, I've seen many different kinds of children, but I see some common themes, too—stressed-out parents and stressed-out children, chronic allergies and illness, anxiety, a short attention span, poor health habits, estranged relationships, insomnia in both children and adults, hyperactivity and depression even in preschoolers, a sense of entitlement, disregard for others, a deep lack of self-confidence, and generalized unhappiness. I see childhood obesity and children seeking desperately for something they can't find—something they often mistake for junk food. Many are prone to colds and ear infections. Sometimes they cry for no reason they can understand. I see underachievers who are unable to pay attention. I see anger, sadness and isolation, and families who have forgotten how to be together in the same room—who can barely look each other in the eye.

Our children are all at risk of trudging through their lives on automatic pilot, fueled by fake food, addicted to junk food, mesmerized by video screens, and tied to texting.

Not coincidentally, these problems occur in families that have strayed pretty far from the way I believe we are intended to live. Their diets are full of artificial substances masquerading as food. They don't exercise. They rarely get outside in the fresh air and sunlight. Some days, they barely speak to one another. They follow the rules society has set out for them to follow, but the spark within them is faint.

My goal is to restore that spark.

There is a link between what children eat and how they develop, behave, and interact with the world—in my work, this is as obvious to me as a child's eye color or height. My goal as an organic nanny, and with this book, is to help you raise your children to be not just healthier and happier than they are right now, but also to be kind, generous, thoughtful people who radiate gratitude, confidence, and intelligence. I believe all children can benefit from the dietary and lifestyle changes I help my clients realize. This book will show you how to lay a strong foundation, put your children on a more natural track, and give them a childhood worthy of remembrance—a childhood that is, perhaps, a little bit better than the one you experienced.

As you look at your own children, no matter whether they are infants or toddlers, tweens, or teens, what are the problems you are experiencing?

What do you envision for your children's future?

Who would you like them to become?

I'm not just here to help children. As a parent, do you find yourself struggling just to get through the day? Are you stressed, cranky, exhausted, frustrated, even depressed? Do you wonder if you are doing everything right for your children? Do you *know* you aren't because you are simply too tired at the end of the day to play June Cleaver?

You don't have to be June Cleaver—but you can be a better *you*. I can help you to replant your own two feet on the ground, as well as the feet of your children. This book is about kids and mothers and fathers and even pets, but to a large extent, the mama keeps the family together, so this book is for *you*. I can help you guide your children better, with less stress and anxiety, and I can help you take better care of yourself, too. Let's get back in the natural world where we all belong.

My History

She listened from the heart.

My grandmother was a petite, bright-eyed Cuban named Evangelina, descended from gypsies, and the greatest healer I have ever known.

We called her Tata. She was a pediatric nurse at a Cuban hospital during a time when it was nearly impossible for a woman to hold such a position, but she also practiced the wisdom of her Cuban ancestors with folk remedies and the kind of common sense that cuts through the confusion and goes straight to the heart.

As a child, I marveled at her almost magical intuition about children. She could always tell what had to be done. I watched as she transformed fresh whole foods and herbs into teas and poultices that helped and healed. I listened as she spoke just the right words to diffuse anger or rekindle affection. I helped her plant gardens and cook meals for the whole family, and I wondered at how she kept our family together and could always help to heal other families, bringing them together, too.

Most of all, Tata always knew what to do and what to say to an anxious child or to a worried mother. She called it "listening from the heart." She forged my destiny as a caregiver and I was her apprentice as far back in my childhood as I can remember. Her gift—a gift she passed along to me—is at the heart of this book.

Much of my philosophy about how children and families should live was formed early in life. My family was forced to leave Cuba during the Cuban revolution. My parents and Tata, connected for generations to the Cuban soil, suddenly found themselves uprooted. They moved to Miami, where I was born, but throughout my childhood, as my parents yearned for their home country, we moved to Puerto Rico, the Dominican Republic, Haiti, and South America.

My older brother Frank and I felt like gypsies, but our nomadic lives always had a constant: Tata, who put down literal roots wherever we went, planting gardens and seeking out the natural remedies of each culture and climate. I learned early how important it is, especially when you don't have a literal home, to make a home wherever you go by connecting with the Earth.

My family wasn't wealthy and we weren't privileged, but I understood what it meant to stand with bare feet in the soil, to rub a healing herb between my fingers and breathe in the green scent, to brew leaves and flowers into a pot of tea, to eat from the garden and let the cycles of the seasons govern my playtime and sleeptime. What I saw, from my naive childhood perspective, were communities of people living close to the Earth, in harmony with the seasons, eating real and whole food, spending time outside, working hard, helping each other in hard times, and because they didn't have many of the so-called conveniences that tend to distract people from one another, standing together and staying together and looking one another in the eye. I didn't know any other way to live.

As a child, I didn't eat processed food—there was no processed food available to us—and I rarely needed medicine or a doctor. I never took vitamins. I ate well, I played hard, and I spent a lot of time outside in the fresh air and sunshine. It was all very natural . . . organic. Tata showed me the remedies I could take from the garden, and she taught me gratitude for gifts from the earth, the family, and the community. I couldn't imagine spending a day staring at any sort of screen, or taking the little we had for granted, or talking back to the adults in my life (well, maybe just a little . . .).

Wherever we moved, in each new place, Tata knitted us into the community by reaching out to children and caring for them all as if each one was her own. She radiated love and healing power. Mothers and children gravitated to her. When a neighbor's child was sick or injured, Tata's patient voice and gentle hand soothed and healed. I remember waking up in the middle of the night and tiptoeing out of my room to peer out into the main room at Tata, counseling a worried mother who had knocked on her door to bring her a sick baby wrapped in a coat. Or she would go to them, holding a sick or injured child against her heart to listen. She never refused a request. Healing was her life and her divine mission.

Although Tata never charged for her services, the love and service she handed out so freely always flowed back to her and she had everything she needed. Relieved and appreciative parents would mow her lawn, paint her house, and provide other chores to give back something in gratitude. I learned so many lessons from my Tata—the importance of community and of a firm and secure foundation, of a routine that a child can rely on, and most of all, the lesson that the earth contains everything we need.

Tata was part of what I later came to see as a great circle of love that pulses and flows with the rhythm of giving and receiving, generosity and gratitude, a circle that revolves along with the seasons as well as the life cycle. At the heart of the circle were the hundreds of children my Tata nurtured. A child mattered more to her than the richest or most powerful adult, and certainly more than work or money or recognition. To her, every child was worthy of reverence. I still live by that credo.

Throughout this book, I bring you Tata's wisdom, coupled with my own. What I've learned from Tata is how to listen for those answers; to really listen to a child who is sick or unhappy or having trouble communicating, and to find the remedies—whether whole foods, natural cures, or behavioral lessons—that will actually make a difference in that child's well-being. I've used these lessons in my work as a nanny, and also in my life as a stepmom, or what I prefer to call a bonus mom, to two beautiful children. I still believe Tata is with me, helping me when I need guidance and teaching me to listen from the heart in my own way to every child that comes into my life.

Your Child's Life

Although progress is often a good thing, there is much to be said for the old ways, and with Tata's help, I want to help you remember the wisdom of your ancestors. For thousands of years, children have lived and thrived on a diet of whole organic foods, fresh water, exercise, sunshine, healthy sleep, close-knit families and communities, and a life in tune with the natural cycles of the Earth.

These children and families certainly had issues, especially those related to lack of the advanced medical care we enjoy today. On the other hand, they also lived free of many of the diseases of modern life—such problems as hyperactivity, attention deficit disorder, depression, obesity, and that chronic sense of entitlement so many kids have today. When you live in sync with the natural world and your survival depends on sticking together as a family and a community, when your only food and medicine comes from the soil in your own backyard, and when you don't have much more than you really need to live a simple life, many health and behavior problems just don't occur. Our lives of excess and privilege have spoiled us in more ways than one—we eat too much, we forget what real food tastes like, and we take our easy lives for granted; and our children are restless, unable to concentrate, and in many ways, unappreciative of their privileged lives. This leads to family fragmentation, chronic illness, behavioral issues, and, I believe, a deep sense of restlessness and unhappiness in us all.

But a more natural life is still available to your children. You can have the best of both worlds—our advanced medical care, conveniences, and technology *and also* a sense of reverence for life, a palate that appreciates real whole food, and a commitment to community and family. Families today have the opportunity and the luxury to embrace the best of both worlds. Isn't it a shame not to live that way?

Of course, these days, to live a more natural life that feeds rather than depletes children isn't easy. In some ways, you will be going against the grain of modern society, where fast food, television, cell phone and computer addiction, chemicals in our food and living environments, rebellious attitudes, and easy fixes are the norm. But at what cost do we surrender our children to the temptations of a toxic world? Childhood obesity has more than tripled in the past thirty years, according to the National Center for Chronic Disease Prevention and Health Promotion. If that isn't a wake-up call that we are collectively doing something wrong when feeding our kids, I can't imagine what is. In addition to food, I see children immersed in environments that also drain health away—environments isolated from real human contact, families who don't communicate, feelings of inadequacy and hesitation and fear.

Your children can have a better life than the one that the twenty-first century hands to them. Research studies now offer hard evidence to prove that what we are eating and how we are spending our time is hurting us, both physically and mentally. I've learned why whole foods nourish, whereas processed foods deplete. I've learned why dairy products may not be as good as we think they are. I've learned about the damaging effects of staring at a screen all day instead of talking to real people, face to face. I've also learned a lot about why children need fresh air, communication, structure, community, and a relationship with nature. Our ancestors knew this by instinct. We may have lost the instinct, but we can relearn what nature has been trying to show us all along.

But I believe it begins with food. Food is the first offering of mother to child, and it is the primary reason families come together every day. Food can work miracles, or create disaster. Food is the basis for what can lift up children to become the very best possible version of themselves—or can keep them down beneath a low ceiling of underachievement and self-doubt. It's never too late to get healthier, and it's definitely never too late to help your children form better habits. I don't care if they are infants or getting ready to leap out of the nest. You can start fresh today, no matter what their age. Make small changes with no guilt, and change will come more easily than you ever dreamed. The industrial food system is engineered to tempt us all, but there is a better way. I'll lead you through it.

In this book, I share my secrets for giving children the gift of a better life. Each chapter provides a framework to help you begin the transformation in your own home, with step-by-step instructions to take you from where you are now to a more organic existence tied to the natural cycles of the Earth, but I'll show you how to do this at your own pace and based on your family's needs. No guilt!

I suspect most busy mothers could use an organic nanny, but not everybody can afford one, and that's why I've written this book—to be your support as you navigate through the sometimes treacherous waters of parenting in the modern world. With each step, I'll be right there with you, and I'll show you what the Earth has to offer you in the way of help and nurturing.

As your personal Organic Nanny, I will take your hand and lead the way. We're going to get reacquainted with the real stuff—genuine, whole, and organic food, the way nature made it. I'll show you how to buy it, cook it, serve it, even grow it. I'll help you seduce your family with it, and gradually win them over. I'll help you get the junk out, the chemicals out, the negativity out—and the sweet, delicious, juicy, beautiful stuff in— into your home and into your children.

We'll go to the market. We'll visit produce stands. We'll learn how to choose the right foods at the grocery store. And we'll take the children along, too, so they can learn what real food really is. It's going to be fun. Then, we'll move on to your home, your family, and *you*.

The Organic Nanny Promise

I'm committed to bringing more life, love, and peace to your family, and that is why this book is my gift to you. Let it be your guide to cleaning up your child's life and restoring health and vitality. In this book, you'll learn how to:

- Wean your family off processed food
- Give noxious processed sweeteners the boot for good
- Reclaim your natural-born right to eat whole grains, instead of processed white flour stripped of its nutrients
- Relearn how to eat real, whole foods and embrace the glory that is Mother Nature's gift to us all: the plant kingdom
- Embrace a life-affirming, passionate, cruelty-free lifestyle by phasing out industrial feed-lot and factory-farmed meat and toxic dairy products from your family's diet
- Get toxins and chemicals out of your personal care products and cleaning supplies
- Gently heal your family with natural remedies, when appropriate
- Take care of yourself so you can best take care of your family. I'll remind you how!
- Make gratitude, respect, and reverence for life a way of life in your home
- Communicate with your kids in a language you all understand by learning to listen and empower children to trust their own inner voice. You can learn to trust yours, too!

CHAPTER ONE

Food, L.O.V.E., and Healing

It's not food if it arrived through the window of your car.
—*Michael Pollan*, from *Food Rules*, rule #20

Children whose problems aren't recognized
become problem children.
—*Marcelene Cox*

The Power of Food

I could tell right away that Harry was a bright little boy with a lot of potential, but to his parents, he had become a constant source of stress. Harry was four and was already reading. He liked to talk to adults and had an impressive vocabulary for his young age. He could charm anyone with his dark blond curls and big brown eyes. However, he had also begun to suffer drastic mood swings. After dinner, he became wild, running around and shrieking, breaking things, and refusing to respond to any requests by his baffled parents to please stop. Bedtime took hours and even after he was down, he kept getting back up. Sometimes he still came into his parent's bedroom after midnight, to ask for yet another glass of juice or another cookie. His exhausted mother kept a box of cookies on her nightstand, just in case he demanded one during the night.

In the mornings, Harry was tired, cranky, and refused to eat breakfast. His mother told me that the only thing she could get him to eat was a frosted Pop-Tart and a glass of chocolate milk. When I came to help Harry and his family, I could see they were in trouble. Harry's parents were no longer able to enjoy their brilliant son because he was literally running wild and they didn't know how to calm him down. But I did.

Hannah's parents had a different problem. Their once energetic and rosy-cheeked little girl had grown sullen and sad. She cried easily, at the slightest frustration, and had to be forced outside to play, where she would sit on the front step, chin in hands, until her mother gave up and let her come back inside. She began to have trouble getting along with other children, and told her mother she didn't have any friends. She looked pale and tired, more like an exhausted adult than a normal, healthy eight-year-old.

Hannah was a picky eater. All her mother could get her interested in were hot dogs, macaroni and cheese, and chicken nuggets. At least she was eating, her mother told me when I came to help them. Hannah barely responded to me until I changed her diet.

Food is life. Food is health. Or food can be the source of frustrating behavior problems, debilitating energy loss, even sickness. What you eat, and especially, what your children are eating on a regular basis, is absolutely crucial in determining their health, well-being, and behavior. They are such beautiful beings—and they rely on us for so much.

The good news is that *you* get to decide: What will you feed them?

I get incredibly passionate about children's health issues, and as a nanny, when I come into a home for the first time, I've seen the whole spectrum: from kids glowing with life to those saddled with physical, emotional, and behavioral problems. I get so excited when I see the kids that glow. For many of the others, my heart breaks—often because I see what they eat.

Many of the children I've nannied have been raised like typical American kids, even those with celebrity parents. We are all in a hurry, and healthy food sounds complicated to most of us, especially when fast food and convenience food is so, well . . . fast and convenient. In my experience, the average child, from toddler to tween, eats just a few things most of the time:

- Macaroni and cheese
- Hamburgers or cheeseburgers
- Hot dogs
- Breaded, fried chicken pieces (nuggets, strips, fingers) or patties
- Soda and other sweetened drinks (even energy drinks!)
- French fries
- Ketchup
- Ranch dressing
- Candy
- Packaged cookies and snack cakes
- A select few fruit and vegetables, mostly baby carrots, bananas, apples, and grapes

Does that sound like food to you? From my Organic Nanny vantage point, it does not look like food at all. The foods on this list are extremely limited as well as (except for the fresh produce) extremely high in fat, and highly refined carbohydrates. It is by no stretch of the imagination a healthy diet. It will not fuel a child's energy needs, but it will encourage fat storage, including arterial fat storage. According to the well-known Bogalusa Heart Study, many children already have fatty buildup in their hearts before they reach the age of ten. A similar study of children in a small Iowa town showed that many young children already have risk factors for heart disease. A report presented at the annual meeting of the American Heart Association in Chicago in 2006 further supported the notion that our kids are at risk. This report combined data from multiple studies, revealing that an increasing number of children already suffer from such conditions as high cholesterol and diabetes, which may lead to heart disease. Among these children, many already showed signs of narrowing and hardening arteries. Many doctors are already putting these children on cholesterol-lowering statin drugs!

More specifically, according to a study by the University of North Carolina of obese children between the ages of one and seventeen, 40 percent of obese three- to five-year-olds participating in the project had raised levels of C-reactive protein, and by age fifteen to seventeen, 83 percent of the obese teens had this same inflammatory heart-disease risk factor. Another famous study called the Framingham Children's Study had better news. This study tracked kids through the end of adolescence, and it showed that children who got more exercise had lower body fat when they became teenagers. Children who ate four or more servings of fruit and vegetables every day had lower yearly blood pressure increases. At the end of the study, children who watched the least television had the lowest body mass index number, an indicator of overweight and obesity.

Food is not a panacea, and it is not the cause of every health and behavior problem in children. However, if your child has a health or behavior problem, I believe it is well worth considering how diet can worsen symptoms—or make the situation much better than it is now. And if your child seems to be doing just fine, why wait for something bad to happen? This book is about taking action and creating change to make our families better than they were before—healthier, calmer, happier, more in tune with each other. We *know* a poor diet and lack of exercise hurts any human's health. Changing your family's health habits now could prevent chronic disease that might otherwise be imminent. A healthy diet is one of the most important things you can control about a child's health. This is your chance to give your child the best possible start in life. Are you with me?

In my work, I've seen big differences in health and behavior corresponding to what kids eat, and it is my mission to help families use food as a powerful tool to help tweak health and behavior problems. My experience reflects the conclusions suggested in all the child health studies I've read: The kids who eat more organic, natural, whole plant foods (you know, such as real, fresh fruit and vegetables, whole grains, and beans) tend to be healthier, calmer, and more in control of their behavior. They get sick less often, they have more energy, and they beam. Sometimes, their parents spend a lot of money on that organic, natural, whole plant food, and sometimes they don't, but I am telling you from my own practical experience that the kids with more natural whole foods in their diet, no matter what the price tag, in general do better in every aspect of their lives than do kids eating mostly high-fat, high-starch, high-sugar, high-animal-content, chemical-laden, processed food.

I call the kids who thrive on whole foods "organic kids." These are the ones who never eat trans fats or chemical ingredients, who have the occasional sweet treat but not the ones made with high-fructose corn syrup, and who eat a low-fat, low-sugar, low-refined-flour, low-or-no-dairy-product diet rich in fruit and vegetables.

And guess who makes it happen? It's you, Mamas. And I've got your back.

Organic kids feel better, look better, and work and play better. This is your great opportunity. The door is open and all you have to do is take my hand and walk through it. It's going to be fun and delicious, and it's going to make *you* feel, look, work, and play better, too. Because "organic" is a family affair. And that is the heart of this book.

Addicted Kids

I am gravely concerned with childhood obesity, which has more than tripled in the past thirty years. Today, about one-third of children in the United States are overweight or obese, according to the American Heart Association. However, that is not my only concern when it comes to fake, processed food. The problem with putting all the attention on obesity is that we tend to ignore the diet of all the kids who aren't overweight. We do this at our peril. High-fat, high-sugar, high-starch, processed food also puts our slimmer kids at a terrible risk for behavioral problems.

We all make excuses for it. It's faster. It's easier. It takes less effort and thought. Yet, this argument doesn't really make sense at all. What snacks could be easier to eat, faster to prepare, and take less thought than an apple or a bowl of baby carrots or a handful of raw almonds? Of course, healthful cooking can be easy or complex, just like any cooking, but choosing the best whole food ingredients doesn't necessarily make it more complicated. Besides, the planet provides us with plenty of beautiful, real, whole food, so why do we feel that we must mess with a working system? The answer is more than a little frightening: Processed food is *addictive*. It may even be considered the twenty-first-century gateway drug.

According to a 2009 issue of *Science News*, a study conducted by researchers at the Scripps Research Institute (a nonprofit), presented at the 2009 Society for Neuroscience's annual meeting, explored the addictive qualities of junk food, and the results were pretty disturbing.

In the study, one group of rats was offered nutritionally complete low-fat rat chow. The other group of rats was offered a diet of processed foods such as bacon, cheesecake, and packaged snack cakes. The group of rats eating the junk food quickly developed compulsive eating habits, eating twice as many calories as those eating the rat chow. They became obese. Those poor rats, forced to eat what Americans eat! After less than a week on the junk food diet, the rats also showed much less activation of their pleasure centers, so they kept seeking more food to get the same "high." The results were eerily similar to what happens to drug addicts on, for example, heroin. I wouldn't give such food to a rat, let alone a child.

Even more startling, the rats on the junk food diet endured electrical shocks to be able to keep eating the junk food. Horrible! The rats on the control diet were briefly introduced to junk food, but when shocked, avoided the junk food. They weren't addicted.

Adam, a handsome, strapping teenage boy and the son of one of my clients once told me, "I feel sick every time I eat fast food, but I just can't stop. I always want to go back because it tastes so good." To me, this is exactly like the poor rats enduring electric shocks just to get their junk food fix. This is what is happening to our kids when they eat processed food. The study concluded that junk food was, in many ways, as addictive as heroin.

So yes, processed food may taste good to your kids. It may look delicious. It may be convenient and cheap, and it may refuse to rot in your pantry. But when it goes into your child's body, you must know what it is doing! I believe most parents don't really recognize what these substances do to kids.

Perhaps you've heard of SAD, the acronym that stands for "standard American diet." Health-foodies often use the term to describe a diet high in processed foods, meat, dairy, and sugar. If you ask me, what the standard American diet does to children is our nation's dirtiest little secret. Our bodies want fresh fruit and vegetables and whole grains in their original packaging, but we can't feel those natural impulses anymore because we are too polluted with junk food. All that salt and fat and sugar has dulled our taste buds and brains, so we've forgotten not just how to eat but how to recognize when we are really truly hungry and really truly full.

Every child is different and different people do better or worse on different kinds of diets. Some do better eating vegetarian or vegan and some do better eating more protein but the one diet that nobody seems to thrive on is a steady stream of packaged, processed "food." Our bodies don't know what to do with all those chemicals and modified ingredients. What our bodies understand is the food Mother Nature made for us. But it's not too late. We can turn around and go the other way, even if we are swimming against the tide. If you and your kids are used to processed food, if they are addicted to these chemicals and denatured ingredients and woefully modified products of industrial agriculture and food science, you can slowly but surely coax your body—and theirs— back into balance. Nothing drastic. Nothing too radical. Just a slow shift back in the right direction, for the health and life of your family.

Out with the Bad, In with the Good

Now, I know what you are thinking, Mamas. You are thinking, "This all sounds nice, but I know my kids. They like what they like and they aren't going to want to eat all new food, especially vegetables."

Don't be so sure. Kids are smart. They like to feel strong and energized, and they like to look good, even if they think eating unhealthy food is fun and rebellious. Even if your children are currently engaging in some bad habits, habits are just that—habits—and they can be changed. Kids have instincts about what they need. A friend of mine has a teenager who recently went on a skateboarding trip with a group of friends. For a week, they subsisted on fast food and bologna sandwiches made with white bread. About halfway through the week, they were all sitting on a ledge outside of a skate park in another town, inexplicably exhausted. Finally, one of the boys said, "You know what I could really go for? Some produce."

"Oh, yeah!" they all agreed, and started fantasizing about apples and salads.

The body knows what it needs. We just have to listen, and some kids are actually better listeners than a lot of adults I know. Sometimes, my clients are amazed to find out how easy it is to go back in the right direction. They have ideas about how hard a natural diet would be to sustain, and when I show them how simple it is, they are genuinely surprised.

My client Sybil, a mother of four, is a perfect example. She always said she was "too lazy to cook." When I came into their home to help them through a transition time, however, it was obvious to me that this busy mama wasn't lazy at all. She was a successful entertainment lawyer and she worked constantly. No wonder she didn't have time for cooking! Cooking just wasn't one of her priorities. She always said she wanted the least possible preparation involved in her meals, and she didn't like to try new things. In addition, while Sybil made a good living, with four children to raise, she was on a budget. She didn't like to spend a lot of money on food. I'm sure many moms can relate to that.

But perhaps not surprisingly, as a result, Sybil's four sons drank soda every day, ate candy multiple times each day, and preferred processed, packaged meals and fast food, because that is what they were used to eating. They also got in trouble . . . a lot. One had several run-ins with the law. They all had poor grades and a hard time concentrating. They talked back to their parents and seemed not to know how to contain their energy. Sybil made a lot of excuses for her boys. They were "typical teenagers," she said. They liked their junk food. In fact, Sybil spent a fortune on packaged food and restaurant meals every week because she thought she didn't have time to cook—so much for saving money.

I saw nothing typical about this situation. When I listened to these boys, I heard that they had fallen into a pattern I've seen many times— bad diet can lead to bad behavior.

I decided to see what would happen if I made healthy whole food *convenient* for this busy family. I went through the kitchen and got rid of all the soda and packaged food. I filled up the cabinets with single-serving packages of nuts, dried fruit, whole-grain crackers, and baked chips. I kept the refrigerator stocked with bowls of apples, pears, plums, grapes, and berries, depending on what was in season. I cut up carrots, celery, radishes, and green peppers and put them on trays with containers of hummus dip and salsa. I filled pitchers with fresh juice and I lined the refrigerator doors with bottles of club soda.

For dinner, I showed Sybil how to boil whole-grain pasta, steam brown rice, and sauté vegetables with flavored tofu or lean organic meats in less time than it takes to get take-out. I showed her how to top tortillas with healthy ingredients for an easy on-the-go meal. I showed her how a few simple herbs and spices can make everything taste great. I even encouraged her to let the boys cook. They were, after all, teenagers, and perfectly capable of making their own food.

Surprisingly, when the boys began to cook, the youngest son, Luke, really took to it. He began to cook most of the meals because he enjoyed it so much, and became a food connoisseur of sorts. He had a knack for combining flavors and began to demand only the highest-quality fresh ingredients. I just loved to watch his transformation. As the boys matured and became more interested in their own lives, I saw them change from irresponsible and distracted kids to healthy young men with ambition and purpose.

Can I credit the food entirely? Probably not, but I'm sure it facilitated their optimal development. The last time I heard from Sybil, Luke was applying to cooking schools. Sybil told me that she was stunned to realize that just because *she* didn't like to cook did not mean that her sons would be the same way.

Is there a closeted chef in your family?

Every family is different. Every mama has different inclinations. If you love to cook, then trying new foods may simply be easier for you. If you don't like to cook, that's fine, too. Either way, choose your foods carefully—because children, as much as they may whine or complain about change, *will* follow your lead.

Transitioning Your Own Family

Most of us know that our children could be eating better (and so could we!), but learning how to make the positive changes to achieve that end may seem intimidating. The next few chapters in this book will walk you through the process of transforming your family's health and diet in ways that are sustainable and pleasurable. Let's do a quick run-down of what's to come.

The first step is a gradual detox. Don't worry, Mamas. Nobody is going to be fasting or living on lemon juice with cayenne pepper. No, what I mean by detox is something very different: I mean the elimination of toxic food from your home. When you get the bad stuff out, you make room for more nutritionally sound choices. When kids want candy and all they can find are bananas and peanut butter or apples and almonds, guess what they're going to eat?

However, change is difficult, so gradual is better. Changing your life for the good takes patience and persistence. You don't have to do it all in one day, and in fact, you shouldn't move too drastically because then you probably won't stick with it. Instead, I'm going to walk you through my family detox method step by step, showing you how to reduce or elimi-nate the so-called foods and food categories that may be causing prob-lems for your children's health. The categories are:

1. *Fast food and processed food.* Beware especially of those contain-ing trans fats (including hydrogenated and partially hydro-genated oils), high-fructose corn syrup, and artificial flavorings, colorings, and preservatives. Chemicals in a box, anyone? I'll show you how to reduce the load in Chapter 2.
2. *Sugar.* Beware especially of white sugar and brown sugar (which is just white sugar with molasses and caramel coloring sprayed on it). A little bit of the sweet stuff now and again isn't going to kill anybody, but too much sugar wreaks havoc on your child's health, sending blood sugar on a crazy ride that can directly in-fluence hyperactive as well as depressive behavior. While not all research supports a behavioral link, many studies have suggested that high sugar consumption contributes to hyperactive and ag-gressive behavior in some children and adults, too. Chapter 3 will inspire you to invite natural sweeteners into your life, so your

child can continue to enjoy sweet foods without mainlining more
processed sweeteners.

3. *White flour.* It's completely stripped of its natural jacket of nutrients. It's just pure starch with some chemicals added on, and the
   more you eat, the hungrier you get. Hello, childhood obesity!
   Chapter 4 will help you transition to wonderful nutrient-rich,
   fiber-rich whole grains.

4. *Dairy products.* You heard me, dairy products. That includes
   milk, cheese, and even yogurt (which is also usually loaded with
   sugar and in many cases, artificial colors and binders. Mmm,
   binders . . .). In Chapter 5, I'll show you the evidence against
   dairy, and why you might want to consider limiting your child's
   consumption, or even eliminating dairy from your home.

5. *Meat.* Factory-farmed meat, poultry, and seafood in particular
   are loaded with chemicals, and many of us also have a problem
   with the inhumane treatment feedlot and industrially farmed
   animals experience. A family who eats primarily plant foods
   with only a little bit of organic, free-range or wild-caught meat
   and fish, or even none at all, tends to be much healthier, slimmer, and more energetic, You'll fill back up with life. Get the
   low-down in Chapter 6.

This list may sound daunting, but don't worry—even step one alone
can make a huge impact on your family. The further you go, the better
you'll feel. You'll be establishing the healthiest possible dietary habits in
your home. To help motivate and inspire you, we'll look at the "why" behind these categories, one at a time. Even more important, we'll look at
the "how," as in, "How do you realistically get the unhealthy stuff out of
your kids' life?"

You can customize how you do this to fit your own family. Every
family is unique, so what I want you to do is think about yours and what
you need. But first, you have to stop and think about this for a moment:
What are you feeding your kids? What are they really eating on a regular basis?

Who Are You?

Before we move on, I'd really like you to give this some serious thought. Stand back from your own life for just a moment, and consider the implications of putting your loving mama stamp of approval on things like soda and fried food and processed food filled with chemical preservatives and artificial ingredients. What price do you really pay for that quick trip through the drive-through, that colorful tray of microwavable whatever-it-is, that frozen bag of fried what-nots?

Do you feed your children what they like? What their friends eat? What appeals to them in the grocery store? What is cheapest? What is easiest? What is fastest to pop in and out of the microwave? I would like you to think frankly about this, because the only way to change your reality is to acknowledge what it currently is.

In what areas does your family's diet need improvement? What are your children's dietary weak spots? What are your own—the things you do yourself, so you are likely to excuse them in others? What are *your* habits and patterns?

Do you suffer from a sugar addiction, or are you more obsessed with fatty salty snacks?

Do you binge late at night, or skip breakfast?

Do you eat out a lot, bring home take-out most of the week, or succumb to the drive-through more often than not?

Do you choose healthful whole grains and lean meats but don't get enough fruit and vegetables?

Do you hate to cook, or do you like the idea but you just don't know how?

Have you always wished you could be a vegetarian or vegan, but you just don't think you could ever give up burgers, or you imagine you wouldn't like the food vegetarians and vegans eat?

Consider all these factors as you embark upon your detox, but also know that there are some ultimate truths that will improve any family's diet. If you want to change your children, and I mean really change them—not who they are, not their beautiful essence, but their health, their hyperactivity, their lack of energy, or their attitude—one of the most important things you can do is to get processed, chemically laced, hormone-soaked food out of their lives.

Maybe you will choose to eliminate one category from your home per week, or go even slower and get rid of one food item in each category per month. Maybe you'll need longer than a month. Or maybe you're more the "cold turkey" type.

The pace is up to you, and you don't have to do these in the order I suggest, either. A gradual detox will be easier on your kids, anyway. (They might not even notice!) You also might choose not to eliminate one or more of these food groups. That's up to you, too. You must listen from your own heart and do what you believe is right for your family. I'll do my best to give you helpful information so you can make the best decision.

Then, in the second half of the book, the wonderful part begins. You transform your diet, and you get to watch as your children get healthier, happier, calmer, more focused, and more aware that what they eat and what they do are all a part of who they are becoming.

And that goes for you, too, Mamas!

All You Need Is L.O.V.E.

You know what's out: processed food, meat, dairy, sugar, and white flour. But let's take a sneak peak at the good part—what's in. I want to introduce you to the L.O.V.E. concept now because it is such an integral part of what I teach my clients and how I live my life.

When you are thinking about what to feed your children, your family, and yourself, you only need to remember one thing. It's the Organic Nanny mantra, an acronym that will remind you of everything you need to know whenever you shop for food or order in a restaurant or even choose a bubble bath product for your children or a cleaning product for your home.

All you need is L.O.V.E.

L.O.V.E. stands for four principles that can govern your family life in a way that will best bring out each person's individual, beautiful nature.

It will unleash in your children health, inner peace, reverence for life, and sense of stewardship over body and planet. I will even go so far as to say that L.O.V.E. will help make all the members of your family into the people they are meant to be on this Earth.

This is what L.O.V.E. stands for:

L: Local
O: Organic
V: Vegetable-centric, vegetarian, or vegan (your choice)
E: Environmentally conscious

L.O.V.E. is how I proceed every time I enter a new client's home, every time I enter my own home, every time I prepare food for my family, every time I clean anything anywhere, every time I step out the front door. It governs the products I use, but even more important, it governs the way I think and feel and live.

L.O.V.E. Transformation

As you and your children live more and more in tune with L.O.V.E., you will begin to notice magnificent but subtle changes. You will all become more sensitive, in the most wonderful ways. You will begin to listen, not just to your own body, but to one another, and to nature, and to your neighbors, and to the world.

When you live with L.O.V.E., your body slowly, gently begins to heal from the ravages of bad habits and modern life. You are already getting the junk out. L.O.V.E. helps you put the beauty back inside. The human body has innate healing powers, but we have to get out of the way by treating ourselves with L.O.V.E., rather than chemicals.

And oh, Mamas, your children! You won't believe what will begin to happen to them when you raise them with L.O.V.E. They get calmer, sweeter, more focused. They get interested in the world, in new and unique ways. Their natural caring and compassion blossoms. Their eyes get brighter, their skin clears, and they gain control over their moods, from toddler tantrums to teenage rebellion. They become who they really are.

So join me in this journey. Start making tiny changes today. Whether you are a junk food junkie or already eat a pretty good diet but you could stand to make improvements, let's get started. Whether you are a vegetarian but eat too many processed products or can't imagine a day without your daily meat, you can start inching toward a healthier way of eating.

Instilling new habits, little by little, will build a whole new tradition for your family—a tradition the industrial food system might not champion, but which you will soon discover (if you don't already know) is better for the physical, emotional, and spiritual health of your children. I guarantee it will feel revolutionary—because it is.

Are you ready? Here is what we are about to do:

1. Detox your kids by getting rid of the food that is interfering with the body's natural ability to heal and radiate health.
2. Make over your kitchen with L.O.V.E.
3. Reacquaint your family with real food and relearn how to eat. I'll give you strategies for winning over even the pickiest kids. You'll also get some delicious, irresistible, kid-friendly recipes at the end of this book.
4. Make over the rest of your life—detoxifying your home; remembering how to take care of you; and restoring a natural sense of gratitude, reverence, and intuition in your entire family.

Finally, I'd like to leave you with a few assignments. I'm going to give you a to-do list after each chapter, containing things I'd like you to think about and do during the week. You don't have to do them all, of course, but at least give them a read and a few minutes of consideration. These are the can-do steps that will really start making things happen.

Organic Nanny To-Do List

☐ Consider your family's dietary habits. Make a list of the good habits, and another list of the habits you'd like to change.

☐ One time this week, when you are tempted to watch television or mindlessly Internet surf, step outside with your children. Breathe the fresh air and feel the sunshine or even the rain. Spend at least fifteen minutes outside.

☐ Think about the list of five items to eliminate from your life and consider which you think will be easy for your kids, and which might be more challenging.

☐ Consider your personal values. Could they help you in your quest to get the junk out?

☐ Embark on a reconnaissance mission to the grocery store, or to Whole Foods or Trader Joe's or other natural foods stores. Look at the foods you've never tried. Become more familiar with the health food aisle. What intrigues you?

☐ Get mentally prepared to make a change. The next few weeks will be exhilarating. Get ready to see gorgeous changes in your kids—and in yourself, too!

CHAPTER TWO

Step 1

Eliminate the Worst Offenders from Your Child's Diet

> Fake food—I mean those patented substances chemically
> flavored and mechanically bulked out to kill the appetite and
> deceive the gut—is unnatural, almost immoral, a bane to
> good eating and good cooking.
>
> —*Julia Child*

*J*ennifer, a young lawyer with six-year-old twins Ben and Matt, prided herself on feeding her children a pretty good diet. They ate fruit and vegetables on most days, only ate whole-grain bread and cereal, and limited fast-food consumption to about once a week. However, the boys always looked forward to that one trip through the drive-through.

Patricia, an older mom with two teenage girls, tried to set a good example by modeling good eating habits herself, but often caved in to her daughters' request for the soda they loved. She saw them so seldom that she wanted them to be happy at home. She had no idea what her girls might be eating when they left the house.

Melanie, an art teacher, prided herself on having switched her daughter, the funny, bright-eyed, beautiful four-year-old Gracie, from packaged food to a colorful diet of healthier organic food. In fact, Gracie's friends at preschool sometimes teased her because the snack her mother sent with her to preschool was often edamame. However, when I was her nanny, Gracie admitted to me that she chose playmates according to their more-desirable (in her mind) lunchbox offerings. She once told me, "I sat next to Sydney today at lunch because she had Doritos and Oreos!" Gracie was getting her junk food fix at school.

All these mothers are doing a good job, but when I came to work for each of them, they knew they had room for improvement. However, they weren't sure where to start or how to make a change, especially with such strong-minded children who loved fast food or junk food, or who were so clever at scoring it.

That is why the first step in your journey with me will be to work on the processed and fast foods that are so detrimental to your children's health. But don't fret! I won't demand you immediately ditch these easy, pleasant foods from your children's life. You'd surely face mutiny! Instead, let's start where you are, and start slowly. Let's start with your children's one worst thing—their weak spot. Let's concentrate on just one junk food or fast food that your family just can't help but eat. Just pick one. That's all I ask right now.

Think about your children: what they eat, what they prefer, and their dietary habits, both at home and away from home. What's the worst thing, the most *obvious* thing you see? Which is the one thing that nobody has to tell you is a really bad idea, but yet, there it is? (Don't be embarrassed; we all have one!)

Maybe it's soda or energy drinks, candy or chips, or overprocessed convenience foods. Maybe it is a time: the starving after-school binge, or the late-night sugar run, or the weekend fast-food bonanza. Just pick one. The worst one, but just one. Let's start there.

This is the beginning of your transformation. I don't want to overwhelm you with a new diet; we're just tweaking your present diet. Changing your child's or family's one worst habit will make a *big* difference.

Even if you never do anything else, you'll be headed in the right direction. This change matters.

De-Junking Your Children

Let's talk about why it's important to de-junk your children.

Kids have a lot of reasons for loving junk food. They see it advertised on television. Their friends eat it. And, because of the careful chemical formulations, junk food has an easy, appealing taste. As I explained in the last chapter, it's also addictive.

Coaxing kids raised on junk food to make better choices is already a challenge, but even kids raised on the good stuff will be tempted to eat what their peers eat. It's just the way our society works right now, unfortunately.

Yet, junk food is the very food that is causing health and behavior problems in our children! Many studies support this notion. A study published in 2003 in *Pediatrics* examined the effects of fast-food consumption on energy intake and diet quality in 6,212 children between the ages of four and nineteen years old. The study followed the children for several years during the 1990s, looking for associations between fast-food consumption and overall dietary quality. The study found that children who ate fast food consumed more calories, more fat, more carbohydrates, more sugar, more sugar-sweetened beverages, less fiber, and fewer fruits and nonstarchy vegetables than did children who didn't eat fast food. The study concluded that consumption of fast food among children in the United States has an adverse effect on dietary quality "in ways that plausibly could increase risk for obesity."

But obesity isn't the only potential problem. Results from a Bristol University study called the Avon Longitudinal Study of Parents and Children, published in the *Journal of Epidemiology and Community Health*, showed that British toddlers who eat more chips, cookies, and pizza before the age of three have a lower IQ five years later, compared with kids who ate healthier diets with more fruit, vegetables, and home-cooked foods. The study allowed for the influence of a home environment conducive to learning, to eliminate that influence. The researchers suggested that because good nutrition is crucial in the first three years of life when the brain is developing at its fastest rate, children who eat too much fat, sugar, and processed food don't get the vitamins and nutrients they need for optimal brain development.

The effects certainly don't end in toddlers. I've read about many studies that link a diet of junk food to emotional problems, from attention-deficit/hyperactivity disorder (ADHD) to antisocial behavior. Several studies have looked at what happens when junk foods are removed from juvenile detention centers or prisons. When the researchers replaced junk foods with healthier foods in these settings, there was a reduction in violence and antisocial behavior. One study clearly showed a reduction in behavior problems with the addition of more omega-3 fatty acids in prisoners' diets (the kind of healthy fat in walnuts, flaxseed, and fatty fish).

I believe the evidence is overwhelming: Junk food hurts kids!

Of course, your kids will always be exposed to junk food in the world, but particularly when they are young, they spend most of their time eating at home. Home is where they will form their habits, preferences, and fond food memories. So, for now, don't worry about what your children are doing out in the world. You can't follow them around every second if they are in school. Instead, focus on what you provide at home, and how you model good eating behavior. What kids learn at home, they often return to as adults, even if they make every effort while younger to sit next to the kid at school with the Doritos and Oreos. This is your chance to make a true impression, one that could last a lifetime.

Phase It Out

How do you start? You can't just throw out all the junk at once and expect to call it a day. Anyone who has children, especially strong-willed ones such as Gracie, knows that it probably isn't going to work. Instead, it's time to ease off the processed food and junk food, in order to eventually eliminate it. Do it too suddenly, and everyone will notice—and rebel! Do it gradually, bit by bit, slowly replacing the bad stuff with better stuff, and your children may not even notice. Or you might find that as you gradually retrain your children's taste buds, they actually start to prefer real food to the pale substitutes they think they prefer.

Let's go back to that one worst thing. Is it the soda? The cookies? The processed chicken nuggets? Whatever it is, gradually begin to replace it with an upgraded but similar food item. Let's look at some examples:

- If you have a pack of soda swillers, keep a pitcher or bottle of fresh, 100% fruit juice in the refrigerator at all times, along with bottles of club soda. Show kids how to mix juice and club soda in a glass over ice, about half and half. Try different juices to find your kids' favorite flavors.
- If your kids love fried food such as French fries and chicken nuggets, try baked versions, which are much lower in fat. Slice up a whole potato, spray with cooking spray, sprinkle with salt, and bake at 400°F for 20 to 30 minutes, or until crispy. Dip raw chicken tenders into beaten egg and roll in seasoned bread crumbs. Bake along with the fries for about 30 minutes, or until no longer pink in the middle (time depends on how big your chicken pieces are). Serve with some berries or apple slices, and you've got a delicious home-cooked meal that resembles fast food!
- If sweets are the weak spot, keep a bowl of easy-grab fruit on the counter and fresh cut-up fruit in the refrigerator. Make homemade trail mix with almonds, peanuts, raisins, dried cherries, and dark chocolate chips and put it in resealable plastic bags for easy snacking, or buy boxes of raisins and packets of peanuts. Also try high-fiber, low-sugar granola bars; whole-grain cookies; and fruit leather. If it's available and easy to grab and sweet, your children will probably go for it.
- If crunchy salty snacks are your children's weakness, keep baked potato chips, popcorn, and flavored mini rice cakes in the cupboard.

Of course, I make it sound easy, but I recognize that upgrading the processed foods your kids love is actually pretty difficult, just because processed food is such an easy (but dangerous!) habit. It feels as if you are going against the mainstream, and that makes some moms and kids uncomfortable.

However, more and more mamas are choosing to lean more toward whole foods and away from the processed junk, so it's getting easier. The tide is changing. Healthier snack options and fun foods are even more available. Plus, so much of what we eat is from habit, so take heart. When you get into the new habit of making something simple—apples and peanut butter, popcorn, celery and carrot sticks with hummus—then it becomes part of your life. It doesn't feel hard anymore, and junk food actually starts to taste like, well . . . junk.

So spend a week or two just concentrating on that one thing you want to eliminate from your family's diet most of the time—the soda, the chips, the sweets, the fried stuff—whatever it is. Focus on that, and you are on your way in the right direction.

The Big Bad Three Ingredients to Avoid

Once you've got a handle on the one thing you want to change, you can start looking around at the rest of your child's diet and making little upgrades and tweaks. There are some easy ways to do this. I'm not asking you to give up all processed and junk food immediately. Some packaged and processed foods and even fast foods are much better choices than others, for example.

However, there are three big ingredients I would very much like you to ditch, right now, and forever more. If you can handle it, just throw them out. Do it while the kids are at school, if you have to.

These three ingredients are your priority. They are easy to spot on a food label, and they have no place in a healthy diet or a healthy child. While you can argue with me about some food items, I won't take "maybe" for an answer on these three. Are you ready? They are:

- Trans fats, including hydrogenated and partially hydrogenated oils
- High-fructose corn syrup
- Artificial anything, including flavors, colors, and preservatives

Just Say No to Trans Fats!

A lot of studies have demonstrated that trans fats harm health. That's why the government now demands that trans fat content be disclosed in foods. However, trans fats do more than skew cholesterol levels. They can also influence mood. In one alarming study, scientists looked at trans fat consumption in the diet of over twelve thousand people. People who ate the most trans fats showed up to a 48 percent increase in depression, compared to those who didn't eat trans fat at all! This research was done in Spain, where trans fat consumption is much lower than in the United States—but even that small amount of trans fat in the diet made a pretty sizeable difference in those subjects' susceptibility to depression! Even more compelling, people in the study who consumed more olive oil and other plant-based fats showed fewer symptoms of depressive behavior. I highly recommend that you ditch the trans fats and use olive oil whenever you can instead. Kids have enough hurdles and challenges these days. They certainly don't need dietary-induced depression.

But wait—does this mean you have to throw out all those bags of snack foods and all that stuff in your freezer? Let's consider why I'm asking you to do something so drastic.

Trans Fats

Trans fats are fake fats. Or, to be more precise, they are vegetable oils subjected to a chemical process that adds hydrogen, changing the molecular structure so the fat resembles a hard fat like lard or butter, rather than its original liquid vegetable fat form. This is how margarine stays solid at room temperature. Adding hydrogen increases the shelf life of food so it doesn't spoil as fast.

Trans fats can disguise old processed food so it still tastes fresh even if it isn't, and that's good for the people who sell the food, even if it's not so good for the people who have to eat it. However, the real problem with trans fats are what they do in the body, raising LDL cholesterol levels, which can lead to clogged arteries and heart disease. According to an article in the *Annals of Nutrition and Metabolism*, trans fat consumption causes narrowed arteries that raise the risk of heart problems significantly.

The most significant source of trans fats is processed food. Recently, the government has required food manufacturers to include trans fat content in their products on the label, making these noxious fake fats easier to identify. You can also tell if a product contains trans fat by looking at the ingredients list. If it says anything about hydrogenated or partially hydrogenated oil, that is trans fat.

Instead, include more healthy plant fats in your child's diet, such as the fats in nuts, flaxseed, avocados, and wild-caught fish. Leave the chemistry experiments for science class.

High-Fructose Corn Syrup

The corn industry tries to make us feel so silly for worrying about high-fructose corn syrup. "It's just corn sugar," they state. Hmm. Well, not exactly. The evidence is definitely mounting that high-fructose corn syrup, or HFCS as it is often called, is definitely not your average sweetener. You might be able to argue that it is pure coincidence that the introduction of high-fructose corn syrup into processed foods about forty years ago also marked the year when obesity rates in the United States suddenly started to rise rapidly, from about 15 percent of the population in 1970 to over a third of us today, when Americans consume an average of 60 pounds of high-fructose corn syrup every year.

However, coincidence or not, a 2010 study published in a journal called *Pharmacology, Biochemistry and Behavior*, from psychology researchers at the Princeton Neuroscience Institute, reported the results of two separate studies designed to determine whether high-fructose corn syrup was the same as other sweeteners. Both studies seem to indicate that the chemically derived sweet stuff really is something entirely different.

In the first study, two groups of male rats were fed regular rat chow, along with water sweetened with either high-fructose corn syrup or regular sugar. The sugar water was at a concentration equal to the sweetener in soda. The high-fructose corn syrup water was at a concentration just half that of a typical soda.

Even so, the rats drinking high-fructose corn syrup gained significantly more weight than did those drinking sugar-sweetened water.

The second study compared rats fed a rat chow diet only, to rats that also received high-fructose corn syrup. Scientists monitored both groups for weight gain and changes in body fat and triglyceride levels over six months. The HCFS rats didn't do very well at all. In fact, the rats gained 48 percent more weight than the rat chow rats did. They also gained significant belly fat and had much higher circulating triglyceride levels.

Sugar and high-fructose corn syrup both have about the same number of calories, so what could be causing the difference? One theory is that the fructose molecules in HCFS are not bound together with a glucose molecule, as they are in regular sugar (sucrose). That means they are absorbed by the body more quickly, without the extra metabolic step necessary to break the fructose-glucose bond. Another theory, which could be related, is that while sugar tends to be used first for energy or to store glycogen in the liver for future energy, and is then only stored as fat after these needs are met, for some reason high-fructose corn syrup seems to bypass this process and is stored directly as fat.

Is it because HFCS is a manufactured chemical rather than a natural sweetener from sugar cane or sugar beets? Likely, scientists say. I say, if Mother Nature didn't make it sweet, than who are we to think we can do better?

Banning high-fructose corn syrup from your home and advising your children not to consume it in any form just might make a big difference in how healthy your kids are, not to mention how overweight they could become. It's a small price to pay for better health and confidence. Just read the label.

Food Additives

What's an artificial ingredient? Who knows? Food manufacturers don't have to tell you anything about how an artificial ingredient was made or what went into it, as long as the artificial ingredient is on a list of ingredients the government considers to be generally recognized as safe. However, science has generally recognized many common food additives as *unsafe,* even if the studies that show safety risks aren't enough to convince government regulators. Personally, I choose to believe the scientists.

For example, aspartame, the artificial sweetener in many diet sodas and other diet foods, has the most complaints reported to the FDA's Adverse Reaction Monitoring System, of any additive. According to the Aspartame Toxicity Information Center, aspartame is a neurotoxin. When digested, aspartame breaks down into methanol and amino acids and a few other things. The methanol is absorbed by the body and converted to formaldehyde, which can cause progressive nervous system damage. Although some food and beverage products containing methanol also contain chemicals that prohibit the conversion to formaldehyde, formaldehyde does seem to form with the ingestion of aspartame, and has been shown to accumulate in the organs and tissues of animals when they are given low doses of aspartame. The more you drink, the more it accumulates in your organs. Formaldehyde is a carcinogen.

Another noxious substance commonly added to food is monosodium glutamate, or MSG. Although MSG's reputation as a Chinese food ingredient is fairly well known, it is actually a widespread additive in processed food and in almost all fast food. MSG is an excitatory neurotransmitter and has been associated in studies with obesity, lesions in the hypothalamus, and many other neurological symptoms that go far beyond that post–Chinese food headache so many people complain about. Studies also link MSG to hypothyroidism in rats.

Nitrates and nitrites, added primarily to preserve processed meat products such as bacon, sausage, ham, and deli meats, prevent the development of botulism in cured meat. However, they are known to cause cancer because, when digested, they form nitrosamines, which promote cancer cell growth. The USDA tried to ban sodium nitrate in 1970 because of its links to colon, stomach, and pancreatic cancer, but the meat industry prevailed and the ingredient remains legal.

Why put all this stuff into our food? It's not the natural way to live or eat or feed our children. The simple foods we already know come from the Earth and are safe to eat are the best foods for our children. So please, read the labels of foods in your cupboards and fridge, and if they list any of the following carcinogenic and/or neurotoxic ingredients, please work on getting those products out of your house as soon as possible:

- Acesulfame-K (artificial sweetener)
- Aspartame (artificial sweetener)
- BHA (preservative)
- BHT (preservative)
- Brominated vegetable oil (BVO)
- Monosodium glutamate (MSG)
- Potassium bromate (bleaching agent)
- Propel gallate (preservative)
- Sodium nitrate (preservative)
- Sodium nitrite (preservative)
- Many artificial colors, especially the five linked with cancer: Blue 1, Blue 2, Red 3, Green 3, Yellow 6

The Processed Food Spectrum

When you first start to eliminate processed foods, you may feel a bit of panic: How will you have time to make everything from scratch? What about when you are in a hurry? What if you are just too tired or can't, for the life of you, think of what to make instead of simply opening the freezer and nuking a box of something you know your children will eat?

I understand, and please don't worry. This is not an all-or-nothing situation. It's easy to say, "If it's processed, don't eat it," but I live in the real world, too. Sometimes your children just really want a bag of chips or a packaged cookie, and it feels easier to hand it over, rather than try to whip up something from scratch when you're in a rush or they're hungry *now*.

Plus, most mamas I know have the thrifty gene. You don't want to just throw into the trash all that food you already bought. What a waste, right? Not to mention the fact that when your kids see bags of chips and cookies in the trash, they might just start a mutiny.

Instead, here is a plan to phase out the bad stuff, softly, sweetly, gradually, as easy as 1-2-3:

1. Use it up.
2. Upgrade it.
3. Phase it out.

For example, maybe your family's weakness is soda. First, use it up. Don't throw it away. If people want to drink it, including you, then just let it go. At some point, all the soda will be gone, and that will be your opportunity to upgrade it.

Upgrade the HFCS-sweetened soda by replacing it with a natural soda that is HFCS free. Many natural foods stores, and even regular grocery stores with natural food aisles, carry sodas sweetened with only real sugar or even fruit juice concentrate. Stick with this for a while. It's still soda! Let everybody get used to it.

Then, try occasionally "running out" of soda altogether. Oops! Sorry, kids! This is how you phase it out, while still upgrading yet again: Offer a club soda–juice mixture as a replacement. Grape juice with club soda is really pretty tasty, but your kids may never know that if you don't give it a try. If they've gotten used to natural soda, they can get used to club soda with juice.

Finally, phase out the soda altogether. Just buy it once a week, then once every two weeks, then once a month, then . . . who even remembers you used to have soda in the house? Pass the grape juice . . .

You can use this same process to tackle addictions to chips, cookies, even candy. Run out, try a healthier packaged version, try the occasional homemade version, and just keep going as well as you can. So many healthier versions of junk foods are available that can make this step-by-step approach much easier than going cold turkey. You just have to be willing to break out of your old habits and try something new. If you buy it, and it's the only choice, your family will eat it, especially if it really does taste good.

For example, here's a nutrition comparison between a fast-food cheeseburger and a veggie burger. Granted, a veggie burger is also processed;

My Favorite Organic Nanny Purse Snacks

Remember Mary Poppins and her magical carpet bag? I love my Mary Poppins bag! Everything in my purse is useful, just like the lamp and mirror in her magical bag. I started calling my bag a Mary Poppins bag because one of the mamas at the Central Park playground used to call it that—whenever anyone needed or asked for something, from a tissue to a Band-Aid to a snack, I always seemed to have what was needed.

One of the most important things I had in my bag, and that you can keep in your own magical bag (a.k.a. your purse), is a few good snacks. As long as they are free of trans fats and high-fructose corn syrup as well as icky additives and preservatives, then the packaging makes them convenient for travel and isn't so bad every once in a while. These also make great transition snacks at home as you are upgrading and working in more whole foods. These are my favorites:

- Earth's Best Sesame Street Snackin' Fruit Hearts & Rings: delicious finger food snacks made from organic whole fruit and oats
- Apple & Eve Sesame Street Juice boxes: 100% organic juice in fun flavors such as Elmo's Punch, Big Bird's Apple, Bert & Ernie's Berry, Grover's White Grape, and Cookie Monster's Orange Tangerine. Watch your children's faces light up when they come eye to eye with Elmo.
- Annie's Organic Fruit Snacks: all-natural strawberry, cherry, and raspberry flavors
- Revolution Foods Organic Jammy Sammy Snack-Size Sandwich Bars
- Whole Foods 365 Organic Potato Chips: sliced organic potatoes, sunflower oil, and sea salt are the only ingredients, and the chips come in kid-size snack bags.
- Whole Foods Organic Seedless Raisins: in purse-size 1.5-ounce boxes
- For kids who can't eat gluten or dairy, I love Nana's Cookie Company. It makes gluten-free cookies without eggs, dairy, or refined sugar, sweetened entirely with fruit juice.

you can't go out to a veggie burger field and pluck one from the ground— a factory made it. But it's still better than the fast-food burger. You can read the numbers.

	In a Quarter Pounder with Cheese	In a Boca Meatless Original Vegan Burger
Calories	510	70
Fat (g)	26	0.5
Cholesterol (mg)	90	0
Sodium (mg)	1,190	280
Sugar (g)	9	0
Protein (g)	48	13

Here are some other processed foods that might be higher in quality than the ones your children have been eating:

- Instead of regular corn or potato chips, try organic corn or potato chips, or sweet potato or vegetable chips.
- Instead of conventional pretzels, try whole-grain pretzels.
- Instead of candy, try organic fruit snacks—individual packs are perfect for your purse or lunchboxes.
- Instead of processed toaster pastries or waffles, try organic varieties made with whole grains.
- Instead of conventional frozen pizzas, try organic pizzas, veggie pizzas, or other frozen organic foods made with whole grains and organic dairy products.
- Instead of movie popcorn, try natural microwave popcorn . . . or pop it the old-fashioned way over the stove, with popping corn and a pot with a lid.

One of my favorite places in the world is Whole Foods. Tata would have loved Whole Foods—it is like a *mercado*, with something for everyone. Browsing the aisles, looking for upgrades to the packaged foods you usually eat is so much fun! If you don't have a Whole Foods near you, look for Trader Joe's or just find the health food section of your local gro-

Water vs. Soda

Tata always believed that water is essential for children. Whenever a child was sick, she always encouraged drinking more water. Water does amazing things for the body. It regulates body temperature, transports nutrients and oxygen into cells, helps flush waste products out of the body through urine and sweat, helps organs absorb nutrients, protects and lubricates joints from knees to spine, and helps all our organ systems work better. Water is good for our skin, muscles, bones, blood, and brain. When kids don't get enough, they can become fatigued, develop headaches and dry skin, suffer from constipation and muscle cramps, even faint from low blood pressure (common in teenagers).

Yet many people walk around mildly dehydrated all the time. Lots of fresh pure water gives you energy and makes you feel clean, inside and out. Why deprive yourself of nature's most precious medicine?

However, when given a choice, most kids choose soda or other sugary drinks over a glass of water. If you get into the habit of making water your primary beverage at home, kids will not only learn to drink it, they'll begin to crave it because they will get back in touch with their own thirst. Serve water at the table with dinner. Keep a pitcher of chilled water in the refrigerator, instead of sweetened beverages. And drink it yourself! Be a water-swigging role model and make water the easiest thing in the house to drink, and you might just convert the ones you love the most.

cery store or food co-op. More and more stores, even small local stores in small towns, are bringing in more organic products, whole-grain choices, and healthier packaged foods. This is where you start, Mamas. When your children still get to open a package or bring something in their school lunch that resembles what the other kids have, it won't seem like such a big deal to make a change.

I don't expect you to eliminate every single processed food forever from your home, but if you practice this three-step approach—use it up, upgrade it, phase it out—or even if you just make it through the first two steps on some items, you'll achieve dramatic improvements in your children's diet—improvements that are virtually painless, and so well worth the future health benefits, as well as the behavior benefits *right now*.

The more you introduce better choices, the more everyone's tastes will slowly mature and develop. Those snack cakes may begin to taste too sweet, or have a chemical aftertaste you didn't notice before. You might also begin to recognize that after you eat them, you feel tired, or irritable, or depressed, and that you don't feel that way after a snack of fresh fruit or whole-grain toast and nut butter. It's amazing how natural foods can make the taste buds more alert and discerning. But start where you are, and take one step at a time. Maybe you just add a plate of fresh fruit to dinner tonight, or put out celery sticks and peanut butter for a snack instead of fried chips.

If your kids weren't always raised on healthy food, it will take some time to find the things they like. Be patient with them, and with yourself. For some kids, if you don't make a big deal about the new foods being "healthy"—if they just think it's dinner—they may be more open to change. You also have to be flexible. Maybe your children will never like broccoli or spinach or sweet potatoes. That's fine. Find something else. There are thousands of delicious, healthy, whole foods out there to try. Even picky eaters can find favorites, if you just keep exposing them to the magnificent variety Mother Nature has to offer us.

In the back of this book and also in the next chapter, you'll find recipes to get you started. Some of them are inspired by Cuban cuisine, which I believe is naturally child-friendly, with sweet rich flavors and very little spice. It's a great way to introduce kids to new flavors they will actually love.

Make the Shift Away from Fast Food

But wait! I'm not done with you yet. We still haven't talked about fast food, and for many families I see, fast food is a major part of life. It makes mealtime easy and the food tastes absolutely delicious to children, so of course it's caught on. Of course, everyone eats it. Don't we?

Of course not. Fast food is a very recent phenomenon particular to the developed world.

As a child, I took for granted that food came from the garden and the greenmarket. Our gardens, no matter where we lived, were always organic just because no one would think of putting chemicals on their tomato plants, squashes, green beans, or strawberries. We shared with the bugs and birds, and every so often, Tata sprayed the plants with soapy water, just to be sure we got our share.

It wasn't until we moved to Miami and I ate fast food for the first time that I tasted anything with preservatives or chemicals. It's also the first time I ever got sick. I wasn't sure what to make of this strange new "food." It's too bad that for many children, junk food is one of their first foods, and their palate becomes trained to prefer it.

Today, more and more families are shunning fast food in favor of more natural choices. Many of them credit the entertaining documentary *Super Size Me* as a primary motivator. In this movie, which I highly recommend you watch with your family, director Morgan Spurlock talks about the "McDonald's Effect"—his term for the influence fast-food places have on children. Believe me, Mamas, this influence is quite purposeful, well researched, and cleverly executed. Fast-food eateries are deliberately designed to be fun play places with bright colors and cool play structures—all the things that seduce children into developing an emotional attachment to the fast-food experience. These companies engineer cheap food that tastes good because of its fat, salt, and sugar, and they pack it in colored boxes with a free toy. All of these sensory impressions stay with children, creating a positive experience and happy memories. I'm not just speaking of hamburger joints—most fast-food restaurants lure children in with the promise of fun and fat and sugar.

Some of these restaurants are now trying to offer healthier choices, due to public pressure, and that may get more families inside the door, but what happens when the kids start clamoring for the fries and cookies and "nuggets" (whatever those are) instead of the healthier options? What child raised on junk food would choose "apple fries" over deep-fat-fried potatoes? And what tired, stressed-out parent won't give in? Because it's just lunch? Because you don't want a battle? Because that's what you always ate when you were a kid?

Family Movie Night

If you haven't already seen *Super Size Me* I recommend you give it a watch, and let your older children watch it, too. It's the fascinating story of a man who decided to see what would happen if he ate only at McDonald's for one month. His vegan girlfriend was horrified! So was he, as he saw how fast food quickly changed his health, energy, and even his mental state. Make some organic popcorn and kick back with people you love.

For older children, such as teenagers, ready for a more moving and disturbing (but true) experience, consider watching the movie *Food, Inc.* together. Be there to answer questions or talk about the issues it raises, and please don't let younger children see it, as it would likely be too disturbing. Some parts are pretty harsh, but it is a message we should all receive: The industrial farming system produces food in a way that is physically and ethically repugnant. You may never shop at the supermarket the same way again!

As adults, we are the first generation to reach adulthood having lived through a childhood where fast food was widely available. Chances are, the smell, the look, and the taste of fast food brings back happy memories. We feel comfort, happiness, nostalgia . . . and we are hooked. *This* is the McDonald's Effect come full circle. The tricks worked on us, so how can we break the cycle? If we are indoctrinated, of course we will be tempted to relive those fond memories with our children in tow.

It's time for an intervention.

Baby Steps

Depending on your family and how you were raised and many other factors, you may have the best of intentions, but you may still give in to the urge for fast food every few days, or weeks, or just every now and again. Wherever you are in your relationship with unhealthy meals, you can slowly begin to turn things around. You can do better. To get you started on the right foot, here are some baby steps that can help you begin to break the cycle and learn how to say, "No—but this is what we *can* eat." Start here. These steps are simple and fun, and there are only two:

Step One: If your children are used to eating fast food on a weekly basis, don't just cut the fast food—that will leave your kids wanting. Instead, gradually shift your family's choices.

Instead of a cheeseburger and French fries, maybe go to Subway or Chipotle and get a sandwich with a few fresh veggies, some baked chips, or a bean burrito with chips and guacamole. Or, keep a stash of low-fat frozen veggie burgers in the freezer at home. A few seconds in the microwave, a whole-grain bun, some natural ketchup (the kind without high-fructose corn syrup), and you've got a pretty good substitute.

Make your own French fries from potatoes sliced, brushed with olive oil, and baked. (For directions on how to create your own homemade "happier meal," see page 48.)

You can still eat some of your favorite foods, but see whether you can do it less. Maybe do it once every *two* weeks, then every three, then once a month. Just as with soda, you can upgrade some of the time as you work on phasing out the bad habit.

Your children may balk at first, but when the substitutes are small and gradual, their palates will have time to adjust. Sandwiches or burritos with milk, water, or juice are fun and delicious, and a big upgrade from a greasy burger, fries, and a sugary drink.

Step Two: Instead of setting your children up to be nostalgic for fast food and junk food, wouldn't it be great if you set them up for nostalgia about beautiful, fresh, organic, real food? Once every week or two, take your kids on a food-related expedition that *isn't* about fast food. Take them along to browse the farmers' market and let them pick out any treat, even from the table of home-baked cookies or the popcorn or slushy stand. Visit a U-pick farm and let them fill up baskets with strawberries, blueberries, tomatoes, or apples. Take them to the natural foods aisle in the grocery store and let them pick out a treat. Pack a delicious homemade lunch and go on a picnic by a lake or in the woods or in a local park. These are the precious times your children will remember forever. *So* much better than recalling all those fun times in the ball pit at McDonald's.

Let Them See

Finally, part of this process is about trust. Trust your kids. They are smart. Sometimes, you just have to get out of the way so they can make the right decision on their own. Seeing children open their eyes and discover what's really going on in the world around them is a beautiful, miraculous experience. If you always stand in the way, they may not be able to see for themselves.

Remember little Gracie, who tried to outsmart her mother's best efforts at sending healthy snacks with her to preschool? I know that forbidding anything usually backfires, but I also like to make my point, so one day when we were in the car together, I drove very slowly into a fast-food drive-through.

"I want chicken nuggets!" Gracie bellowed with all her four-year-old lung power. "Not the square kind, the star-shaped kind! And I want ketchup. And honey sauce. And can I have a chocolate shake, too? Can I? If I finish my nuggets, can I please? I promise I'll finish them all! And I want a pink Barbie toy!"

"You guys need any napkins with that?" chuckled the drive-through attendant.

Gracie was playing right into his hands. "Okay, Gracie," I said, "how about this. I get you what you asked for, but you agree to participate in a little science experiment with me." Gracie agreed. We bought two fast-food lunches—one for Gracie, and one for our science experiment.

When we got home, Gracie gobbled up her meal as I watched.

Organic Nanny Notes

Depending on what it contains, a McDonald's Happy Meal contains between 380 and 700 calories and 12 and 27 grams of fat—the high end of that scale is a cheeseburger Happy Meal with French fries and chocolate milk. These are far too many calories and fat grams for a child. A Happy Meal does not make the Organic Nanny happy.

Then, I told her about the experiment. Real food, I explained, gets digested by our body. If we don't eat it fresh, it will spoil as it prepares to go back to nature. Fake food, however, doesn't rot because it is filled with strange chemicals that make it more like a piece of plastic than a yummy meal.

Gracie nodded, interested that she was being given this very adult information.

"I am going to put this meal up here on the shelf," I told her. "If it is real food, then in a few days, it will be all rotten. If it's more like plastic, then it will probably look the same as it does right now. Let's look at it."

Together, we peered into the box. We opened the nuggets, we surveyed the crispy fries, we examined the toy Barbie. Then we put it on the shelf.

I admit, I had heard about this experiment before. Others have tried it, and I expected the same results. Sure enough, that's just what we got.

The next morning, we discovered that Gracie's cat had found and eaten all the French fries. Yet, she left the chicken nuggets untouched, making us wonder what could have turned a feline carnivore away from this so-called meat.

As for the nuggets, they looked exactly the same the next day. And the day after. And the day after. A week after we put them on the shelf, we threw them away—they were as unchanged as the Barbie doll.

"Would you eat a Barbie?" I asked.

She shook her head vigorously—and went back to the apple she was eating.

If I would have just handed down the harsh rule that Gracie was not allowed to eat fast-food meals ever again, I would have had one rebellious four-year-old on my hands. However, because I let her see, in several ways, why that food wasn't best for her, she came to the conclusion on her own.

During the time I was her nanny, I never heard her ask for fast food again.

Your journey toward a healthier diet may not be so black and white, but trust me: When you begin to clean up your home, your kitchen, and your diet, everyone in your family will begin to feel the positive changes.

DIY Happier Meals

Are your kids totally addicted to the fun fabulousness of junk food in a colorful box with a toy? While some forward-thinking cities and counties (I'm looking at you, Santa Clara, California!) are banning the practice of including toys with fast-food meals marketed for children, you can enact a gentle sort of ban of your own by making homemade "Happier Meals" that are even more appealing than the fast-food variety.

First, go to your local dollar store or other discount shop and stock up on small, inexpensive toys such as mini dolls, toy cars or robots, small stuffed animals, or miniature coloring books and crayon packs. Keep the stash handy but hidden—these toys are only for your very special home-made "Happier Meals."

Next, find a good veggie burger your children like, such as the Original Vegan Meatless Boca Burger. Buy a soft, smallish variety of whole-grain hamburger bun. Add some ketchup made without high-fructose corn syrup (Hunt's carries a 100% natural variety, and Heinz makes an organic ketchup. Both are available in many grocery stores).

Make your own, healthy baked "fries" (see page 234), or if you don't have time for that, add a *small* bag of baked chips or another crunchy snack such as Popchips.

Add an organic juice box—check out the ones by Apple & Eve (see page 39). Or, if your child prefers, add a box of plain, chocolate, or vanilla soy or rice milk.

You could even include a packet of all-natural fruit snacks or a square of natural chocolate for dessert.

Pack it all into a colorful gift bag. Dollar stores often have gift bags and even gift boxes at a very affordable price. Send it to school with your child, and just watch what happens when your child eats a fun, fanciful meal that makes you both happy!

When your kids notice for themselves that they feel better and look better on real food, they will be taking that first important step toward food consciousness, which is to say, they will be taking that first important step toward a healthier life.

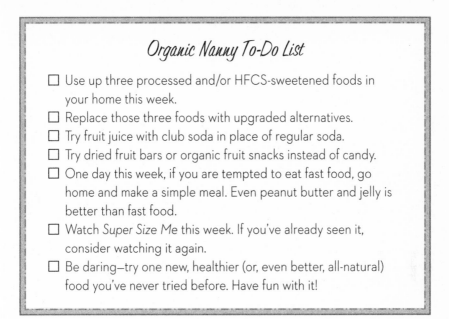

Organic Nanny To-Do List

☐ Use up three processed and/or HFCS-sweetened foods in your home this week.

☐ Replace those three foods with upgraded alternatives.

☐ Try fruit juice with club soda in place of regular soda.

☐ Try dried fruit bars or organic fruit snacks instead of candy.

☐ One day this week, if you are tempted to eat fast food, go home and make a simple meal. Even peanut butter and jelly is better than fast food.

☐ Watch *Super Size Me* this week. If you've already seen it, consider watching it again.

☐ Be daring—try one new, healthier (or, even better, all-natural) food you've never tried before. Have fun with it!

Once you've begun the process of eliminating processed food from your lives, you will begin to feel stronger and more energized and more clear-headed about your food choices, too. That is when you will be ready for the next step. Be ready, because it's a challenging one—but I just know you have the courage and persistence to make it happen!

CHAPTER THREE

Step 2

Sugar Freedom

I eat my vegetables. My favorite is pumpkin pie.
—*Nicole, age 4*

Octavian screamed to the point of exhaustion. The little boy's tantrums seemed so inexplicable, so random, and so unlike the sweet, charming little boy he usually was. Then one day, I made the connection to sugar.

I noticed that an hour after eating cookies or the candy he loved, especially jelly beans or M&M's, Octavian would have a tantrum. This one was set off by frustration. Octavian couldn't finish a puzzle, and out of nowhere, he began throwing the pieces and shouting, and then he was beyond reason. Normally, Octavian could handle minor frustrations. He might not finish a puzzle, but it certainly wouldn't enrage him.

I decided to test my theory. I watched him to see if it would happen again, and sure enough, every day, an hour after a sweet snack, the little guy would have a meltdown. The cat wouldn't stay in his room, or his mother wasn't home soon enough, or I wouldn't let him have another handful of candy.

I sat down with his mother and told her about my theory. The more we thought about it, the more we both recalled numerous times when tantrums were indeed linked to a sugary treat. So, we devised a plan. We threw away everything in the house that contained high-fructose corn syrup or white sugar—bags of candy, cookies, sweet cereal. (We did this while Octavian was napping.) Instead of his usual sweet snacks, we gave him protein-rich treats, such as half of a peanut butter sandwich; a fruit smoothie with protein powder; cottage cheese and carrot sticks; a bowl of oatmeal with cinnamon, raisins, and soy milk; celery sticks with almond butter; or a bag of homemade trail mix with dried fruit and nuts.

The next time Octavian asked for cookies, I convinced him to eat his healthy snack first, and after his snack, he didn't seem to want them anymore. That afternoon, he played happily without incident. His mother was amazed when she came home from work. She'd rarely seen him so calm right before dinner. Over the next few weeks, he occasionally asked for some candy, and once or twice he even cried. However, his upsets were nothing like his former tantrums, and when I explained to him that candy made him sick, he seemed to understand. He must have sensed it himself. "But I want it!" he said once. "I know you do," I told him, sympathetically, "but these peanuts are just as good!"

After about a month, he stopped asking for sugary foods, and when I left him, I hadn't seen a tantrum in months. I imagine he still eats sugar once in a while, but I hope for his sake that he is off the heavy sugar habit for good. Some children do okay on sugar, or so it seems, but others are simply very sensitive to its effects on blood sugar. Octavian was one of those children. Could your child be that way, too?

Is Your Child Already Addicted?

Oh, sugar—sweet sugar. How attached we all are to the stuff that boosts our moods and brightens our days. But my heart breaks for children today. While the whole world denounces sugar and high-fructose corn syrup as unhealthy, they are dangled in front of your child constantly.

Organic Nanny Notes

Processed foods that are high in sugar confuse your child's natural hunger signals, so they eat more than they need or biologically desire. A Harvard study published in the *Journal of the American Medical Association* revealed that overweight adolescents ate 500 calories more on days when they ate junk food, than when they were prohibited from eating junk food. Junk food actually seems to fuel the appetite, even though it is high in calories.

On reviewing the study, one of the doctors I greatly admire, Dr. Mark Hyman, chairman of the Institute for Functional Medicine, wrote, "Like an alcoholic after the first drink, once these kids started eating processed foods full of the sugar, fat, and salt that triggered their brain's reward centers, they couldn't stop. They were like rats in a cage."

Yikes! Let's free our kids, Mamas! When you unshackle children from the heavy chains of high-fructose corn syrup and other processed sweeteners, you set them free to thrive.

Schools have candy and soda machines. Teachers give out candy and cookies as rewards. School parties are basically giant sugar festivals. School lunches contain sugar and high-fructose corn syrup in many of their offerings, not just dessert.

Out of school, it's even worse. Television and Internet advertisements tempt your child with charming images and clever jingles about sugary snacks. Sweetened cereal is advertised as a healthy breakfast, and even seemingly benign foods such as ketchup and yogurt are filled with the addicting, fat-boosting, blood sugar–destabilizing stuff.

We have become a nation of sugar addicts.

The problem is, you can't just give up an addiction out of sheer will power. Your kids need help doing that, and you can provide it. As Dr. Hyman has written, "We blame the fat person. But how can we blame a two-year-old for being fat? How much choice do they have?"

Protein Power

One of the best ways to combat the urge to splurge on sugar is to eat protein. Start out your child with a protein in the morning, every single day, and she will be less likely to default to gotta-have-sugar mode. Protein helps stabilize blood sugar. A little bit of peanut or almond butter, eggs, tofu cubes, veggie or turkey sausages, or mashed white beans on whole-grain toast will begin your child's day on a much more solid footing than will sweetened cereal, white bread with jam, or syrup-soaked waffles.

How Too Much Sugar Can Affect Your Child

Experts recommend that children eat no more than about 100 calories of sugar each day. Yet, according to a 2010 poll in *Family Circle* magazine, the average teenager eats about 34 teaspoons of sugar every day. That's 500 calories' worth! But what if you have a superactive kid who can burn those calories? Is too much sugar still a bad thing?

People used to talk about the "sugar high" that kids would get, in reference to hyperactive behavior. In the last few years, several studies have supposedly debunked this myth by demonstrating that sugar did not have a behavioral effect on some children. In my experience, however, the key to that conclusion is "some." Some children don't seem to suffer a behavioral lapse after consuming too much sugar, but others definitely do. Every person has a unique biochemistry that may or may not involve allergies and sensitivities. Those who are sensitive may be hyperactive or may get depressed, or may swing wildly between the two. Too much sugar can also reduce attention span in some children, and may also depress learning ability. If you have a sugar-sensitive child (like Octavian), you probably already know or at least suspect it.

But sugar causes even more problems. Several studies have demonstrated that the immune system response becomes depressed after subjects drank a sugar solution containing about 20 teaspoons of sugar, or the equivalent of two cans of soda. White blood cells suffered a 50 percent decrease in effectiveness in fighting bacteria, peaking about two hours after the sugar was ingested and lasting up to five hours afterward. One study measured the adrenaline level in children after dosing them with sugar, and in some, it rose to ten times higher than its normal level and stayed that way for five hours.

Yet another study compared a group of preschool children who had ingested a sugary drink (whose sugar content was equivalent to that in a can of soda), with another group that didn't consume any sugar. The sugar group was noticeably more hyperactive and displayed decreased performance in learning. And teachers are giving kids candy in school? Perhaps they don't realize how much they are thwarting their own efforts to teach by making their students less teachable!

Children with attention-deficit/hyperactivity disorder are even more at risk from sugar consumption than are children without that condition. After a dose of sugar, they have a more extreme blood sugar spike than do other children, and they apparently metabolize sugar differently. Normally, a blood sugar rise releases hormones that help regulate blood sugar, but some studies suggest children with ADHD are missing this normal response.

In her book *Sugar-Free Toddlers*, author Susan Watson reports that a juvenile detention facility in Virginia called the Tidewater Detention Homes "found that by significantly reducing just the amount of sugar in adolescents' diets, the rate of antisocial behavior dropped 44 percent. They also found that there were 82 percent fewer assault incidents, 77 percent fewer theft incidents, and 55 percent fewer incidents of refusal to obey requests!" This is a pretty significant indicator that sugar can have a major impact on the behavior of children of all ages.

Sugar also feeds the intestinal bacteria that can lead to digestive problems, and it can contribute to yeast infections and thrush. And we all know sugar can lead to tooth decay and cavities.

Finally, in both children and adults, sugar is one of the most powerful appetite stimulants known. The more you eat, the more your blood sugar spikes, which releases a flood of insulin, which causes the blood sugar to drop, which results in cravings for more sugar. It's a vicious cycle that's very hard to escape. The sugar habit is truly an addictive one.

Now, I love a good cupcake as much as you probably do, but the problem is that sugar used to be reserved for special occasions. When it's a big part of every day, it throws our body out of balance, especially in those who are sugar sensitive. You probably know kids (and adults) who seem to be able to eat sugar and have no problem with it. They are calm, smart, and thin. Even more baffling, they can eat, for example, one cookie, or even part of a cookie, and stop. They might even pass on a plate of cookies if they just aren't in the mood for sweets.

Not in the mood for sweets? What's up with that? To a sugar-sensitive person, that's inexplicable. These children want sugar so badly that it's hard to say no, but you have good reasons to say no, Mamas.

First, think about your own child. Do you think you have a sugar-sensitive little one?

You can spot a sugar-sensitive child by these traits. Is your child (or are you):

- Constantly asking for and craving sweet foods? Children do this because they are so sensitive to that blood sugar roller coaster.
- Unable to stop eating sugary foods once getting started, such as wanting a third toaster pastry or eating a whole box of cookies or a whole bag of Halloween candy? When the pleasant mouth taste overrides a feeling of fullness, a child has lost control of his ability to judge his own appetite. That's a sure sign that you need to step in.
- Always wanting sweets while watching television? Mindless eating is comforting, but when kids eat sugar mindlessly, they can take in hundreds of extra calories while barely noticing.
- Frequently irritable or explosive? Sugar releases cortisol, a stress hormone, which can make some children, especially those who are hyperactive, more irritable. In fact, some studies show that children with ADHD behave more aggressively after eating sugar than do those who behave aggressively without having the disorder.
- Suffering from dramatic mood swings? The blood sugar spikes and drops can translate directly into behavior spikes and drops in some children—sugar-induced bipolar-like symptoms.

I'll Tell You Where to Put the Sugar . . .

Mamas, I will never advise you to use a spoonful of sugar to help the medicine go down. Cut the sugar, and chances are, your child won't need medicine!

But don't dump that sugar in the trash! Instead, I have a much better use for the sugar you have in your pantry. This works for white sugar or brown sugar. Just mix that sugar in a bowl with a little bit of olive oil, and use it as a luxurious body scrub the next time you take a shower.

Scrub your elbows, heels, arms, legs, even your face, and watch radiant smooth skin emerge. Consider it your special mama-pampering beauty secret. As long as you keep it on the outside of your body, sugar will make you glow.

- Overly emotional, crying all the time? Sugar can trigger mood swings, including a feeling of uncontrollable emotions in some people, also likely due to its effects on blood sugar and hormones.
- Depressed? As with emotional behavior and mood swings, sugar seems to make some people feel depressed.
- Having a hard time paying attention or sitting still? As noted earlier, sugar can cause some children to display hyperactive behavior and can cause problems with attention.
- Catching colds all the time or suffering from allergies? This has to do with the depressive effect sugar has on the immune system.
- Overweight? Sugar in all its forms has clear links to excessive weight gain.
- Experiencing frequent ear infections? Again, this has to do with sugar's immune system–depressing effects.

Although it is certainly true that these symptoms of sugar sensitivity could also be caused by other problems, they are certainly red flags for any parent that something is wrong. Cutting out most sources of added sugar in your child's diet is one of the easiest ways to start setting things right again. Don't worry about special occasions for now. Just concentrate on getting that daily dose reduced and eliminated. It may not solve all your child's problems or have as dramatic an effect as it did on Octavian, but what if it did? Isn't it worth trying? I've seen reduced sugar consumption, and in some cases, complete added sugar elimination, make seemingly miraculous changes in children's behavior. It's certainly something to try before resorting to medications such as amphetamines or antidepressants! And even if it doesn't solve every behavior problem, it will most certainly promote better health. A body unburdened by processed sugar is better able to heal because all of the things sugar inhibits in the body are finally set free to do the work they were meant to do.

How to Beat the Sugar Blues

If you think you do have a sugar-sensitive child, or if you simply know that your child eats too much sugar, it's time to do something about it. You don't need to banish sweet tastes from your home. Just be a little stricter about the processed stuff.

Children love sweet tastes, and that is completely natural. You can't fight it. Sweetness itself isn't bad. We are programmed to seek out sweet things as good sources of nutrients, and many whole foods have a sweet taste, complete with fiber and vitamins—fruit, some veggies, maple syrup, and grain-based sweeteners.

It's not even the sugar cane plant that's the problem. It's what we've done to it.

Sugar has a whole-food form, although few people in the United States have probably ever seen it. When I was a child in Puerto Rico, Tata would put a machete in the front seat of her car, drive out to the sugar cane fields, cut down a small bundle, and surprise my brother and me with a seriously tasty treat! We chewed on those sweet, juicy canes, and that was enough. We didn't bounce off the walls, want more and more, or have a crash and need a nap.

For one thing, sugar cane was considered special. It wasn't for every day, the way kids consume processed sugar now. It was a very occasional treat. For another, it was natural, unprocessed sugar in its original form, with all the fiber and minerals and hundreds of other minute plant sub-stances (called phytochemicals—good chemicals engineered by Mother Nature) that have yet to be named. It was a whole food.

But sugar cane bears no resemblance to what most families keep in the sugar bowl or what food manufacturers pump into their lab-formulated, processed products. We've changed the nature of this perfectly innocent plant, until it doesn't even remotely resemble its natural form. Sugar cane goes through numerous processing steps to become the white crystals we know as sugar, and they are far from natural.

One of the reasons why I love Cuban cuisine so much is that it con-tains naturally sweet tastes. However, it doesn't contain the degree of sweetness the standard American diet does. Also, those tastes don't have to come from sugar. Natural sweeteners such as fruit juice, molasses, real maple syrup, brown rice syrup, raw agave nectar, sorghum, and raw evap-orated cane juice add a more authentic flavor than do those soulless white crystals. Once you get used to the rich complex interesting taste of nutritious whole-food natural sweeteners, white sugar tastes like chem-icals. And you'll be set free, and you'll feel more stable and able to begin reducing your overall consumption of sweeteners.

But like every other step in the Organic Nanny detox, you'll find it is easiest to give up sugar if you do it gradually. While some people take the cold-turkey approach (and sweat out the side effects), this can be too harsh for a child.

As with the other steps, first use it up. Don't be in a rush to throw all your child's favorite foods into the trash, unless you have a sugar emer-gency, like Octavian's. In that case, toss away, but not while your child can see.

Then, as the cookies and candy and other sweet stuff run out, up-grade to products containing less processed sweeteners. Natural sweet-eners don't taste exactly like sugar, and your child may not like them as much at first. However, as your child's palate cools off from the super-sweet effects of processed sugar, she will start to appreciate other sweet tastes more.

I've seen this happen many times. Janie was a sweet but fiery seven-year-old redhead, and I was her nanny for a few months while her regular nanny was on a leave of absence. Janie absolutely loved sweets, and I could tell right away that she was sugar sensitive. She would eat cookies until someone took away the plate or the bag, and after a package of candy, she was never satisfied. She always wanted more. She also tended to have mood swings. Her parents attributed this to her fiery hair and Irish heritage, but I had a suspicion her mood swings were related to more than genetics.

First, I began to bake for Janie. Instead of the packaged cookies she was used to eating, I gave her homemade cookies. I began by using raw sugar instead of white sugar, and gradually, with each batch, replaced part of the white sugar with a natural sweetener, such as honey or maple syrup or agave nectar. I also gradually began to replace a proportion of the white flour with whole wheat pastry flour. Sometimes I added oats.

At first, Janie thought the cookies tasted "a little funny." However, when her regular cookies weren't available, my cookies were better than nothing. Pretty soon, she began to request them. Slowly, slowly, I kept tweaking the recipe, adding more whole-grain flour, substituting dried fruit for some of the chocolate chips, adding some chopped nuts, and slowly reducing the amount of sweetener and increasing the proportion of natural sweetener to cane sugar. By the time I left her (and left her mother with my recipe), the cookies were very healthy cookies.

I also began to swap out Janie's candy snacks with fruit snacks and dried fruit mixed with nuts or peanuts. Sometimes, we made our own treats, such as homemade marshmallows or taffy. On some days, I sighed and admitted to Janie that all we had was fruit, but I would cut up a bowl of sweet, juicy fruits and sprinkle them with just a tiny bit of sugar or a drizzle of real maple syrup, and special toppings such as a teaspoon of mini chocolate chips, a little bit of coconut, or a few sliced almonds. She sighed too, but somehow, she made do . . . and ate every bite. She almost brought tears to my eyes the day she actually requested that I make her the "Nanny Fruit."

Over the months I knew Janie, I watched her transform from an unpredictable and moody grade-schooler to a calmer, supersmart young girl with amazing creativity and a passion for her hobbies, which in-

Sweet and Natural

Natural sweeteners to enjoy:
- Agave syrup (agave nectar)
- Honey
- Real maple syrup
- Molasses
- Brown rice syrup
- Sorghum
- Fresh fruits and their juices and concentrates
- Dried fruit
- Unrefined cane sugar (e.g., Sucanat)

cluded jump rope tricks and origami. Where she once became easily frustrated, she now had more patience and was able to accomplish more skilled maneuvers with both her jump rope and her folded paper. Some of this was certainly due to her gaining in maturity. However, my last day with her, she actually sat down and concentrated long enough to make an origami crane for me, and I bet she was able to do that in large part because of her sugar-reduced diet.

You can phase out sugar in just the same way. Simply stop buying every single regular sweet item you normally buy. Try alternatives, both naturally sweetened packaged foods and homemade foods, where you control the ingredients. If you don't like to cook, no worries! There are so many great options now in most grocery stores, and especially in natural foods markets. You can find cookies, cupcakes, muffins, snack bars, granola bars, and cereal that are naturally sweetened or have reduced sugar. Try reserving desserts for the weekend only and replacing sweeter snacks with sugar-free snacks, such as celery with (no-sugar) peanut or almond butter, guacamole or hummus with whole-grain chips or crackers, cups of soup, or a simple piece of fruit.

Here are some other ideas for sweet, kid-friendly foods to keep around the house at all times, prepared to eat and within reach of little hands:

- A bowl of fresh organic fruit on the counter or in the refrigerator. Try apples, bananas, oranges, peaches, nectarines, plums, and pears, according to what is in season (when they taste best!)
- A bowl of freshly washed organic berries or grapes in the refrigerator. Try strawberries, blueberries, blackberries, raspberries, and grapes grown in the United States (they have the least amount of pesticide).
- Packaged snacks in the cupboard. Try dried fruit such as raisins, cranberries, cherries, blueberries, figs, and prunes; fruit leather and fruit snacks (low sugar or naturally sweetened); fruit-and-nut snack bars (try the amazing Larabars for a real treat); and homemade or purchased trail mix with nuts and naturally sweetened dried fruit.
- Boxes of naturally sweetened breakfast cereal, both cold and hot.
- Juice pops and naturally sweetened frozen treats in the freezer. Try individually wrapped Rice Dream Non-Dairy Frozen Dessert Pies, Luna and Larry Coconut Bliss products, and Tofutti Cuties ice-cream sandwiches.

There are so many sweet treats out there that don't contain highly processed sugars. Go to the store and explore. Let your child help pick out treats, and show him how to read the labels to look for the poisons: high-fructose corn syrup and sugar! Whenever you can, steer him toward snacks that don't contain any sweetener at all.

There are a million different ways to make simple sweet treats at home. Here are just a few to get you started:

- Slice a banana and drizzle with maple syrup and naturally sweetened or plain soy milk.
- Freeze very ripe bananas (peeled), then put them in the blender with a little cocoa powder, agave syrup, and any kind of milk (I like coconut milk). Blend to make a delicious healthful milkshake or "ice cream."
- Make a parfait of nondairy plain yogurt with fresh berries and agave nectar drizzled between the layers.

Organic Nanny To-Do List

☐ Use up one packaged food item containing processed sugar and replace it with a similar packaged item that is naturally sweetened.

☐ Try baking your favorite dessert with half the sugar, or if you aren't a home baker, try a new brand of organic, naturally sweetened, store-bought baked goods or baking mix.

☐ Replace at least one sweetened drink per day (soda, fruit punch, even a juice box) with a glass of water, or encourage your child to drink a glass of water first and then see if she is still thirsty.

☐ Make a glass of lemonade with the juice from four freshly squeezed lemons, club soda, and 2 or 3 tablespoons of agave nectar, or more if necessary. Taste until you get the sweetness right, but remember, lemonade should be more tart than sweet.

☐ Do something sweet for your child today that has nothing to do with food. A big hug and kiss? An hour of uninterrupted storybook or coloring time? Going to the park to swing on the swings, cell phone turned off?

- Sprinkle toast with cinnamon and "frost" with honey.
- Serve real maple syrup over whole-grain pancakes or waffles. (Mix with regular pancake syrup to get your child used to the taste first.)
- Try almond butter toast with a light drizzle of agave nectar, maple syrup, or even molasses or sorghum, if your child is adventurous.
- Spread natural (unsweetened) peanut butter in a stalk of celery and top with a line of raisins for the classic "ants on a log" snack.

Freeing your child from sugar's sweet embrace can feel like an insurmountable challenge at first, but it really only takes a week or two to break sugar's grip. Soon, your child will actually be able to taste sweetness in so many other forms, from fruit to sweet potatoes to the natural sweetness in spices such as cinnamon. And remember, moderation is key. For some children, banning something for all eternity is likely to result in rebellion, or at least in resentment. Better to leave the real sugar out there in the world where your child will occasionally encounter it. Let home be a largely sugar-free zone, and reap the health, weight, and behavior benefits. They are significant.

Finally, always remember that life should be sweet—but sweetness shouldn't always have to come from sugar. There are so many ways to add sweetness to a child's life, and most of them involve *you*, not a cookie. Spending uninterrupted time with your child, no distractions, no cell phones, no checking e-mail, is one of the greatest gifts you can give. More than anything else, your child wants your attention, and the more he gets it, the less he might be clamoring for a replacement in the form of sugar. So give your babies some sugar right now! And by that I mean a great big kiss.

CHAPTER FOUR

Step 3

Phase Out White Flour, Embrace Whole Grains

*C*hristopher was a "big boy." At least, that's what his mother used to call him. I suppose you might call him "strapping," but truthfully, he wasn't very muscular or powerful. He was simply very overweight. Christopher was also smart. He liked to talk to adults and he had a remarkable vocabulary for his twelve years. He was interested in what was happening in the world and he always wanted to know the opinions of his parents and other adults, whether about the latest international crisis or some controversial national issue or even the latest nutrition news. He was always coming up with his own ideas for how people should be doing things better.

Christopher also loved toast. I mention this along with the other dominant parts of his personality because he *really* loved toast. He ate white bread toast multiple times per day. He ate it for breakfast with butter, for lunch with peanut butter and jelly, and as a side dish for dinner. He was responsible about his habit—he would take the loaf of bread from the refrigerator, unwrap it, take out a slice or two or three, toast them, put the bread away with the package neatly tied, then put his toast on a plate. He would melt butter in a little dish and brush it on the toast with his mother's basting brush, or he would spread the peanut butter and jelly carefully, cleaning up any messes he made. Then he would sit at the table with a napkin and eat every crumb.

It was hard to be hard on Christopher. He was just so agreeable and well behaved and eloquent! His parents admired him greatly and often talked about how intelligent he was. I agreed with them, but I was concerned. He had to have his jeans specially made because you couldn't buy jeans that short with that large a waist size. He already had quite a spare tire that extended over the top of those jeans on either side. His thighs rubbed together when he walked, and he sometimes complained (always with some embarrassment, and only in private) that he was "chafing." I knew children at school made fun of him, and he laughed right along with them, calling himself fat, but I could see the pain in his eyes.

Unlike many kids his age, Christopher wasn't particularly interested in sugar. I never saw him eat candy or drink soda, and he liked to drink a lot of water. However, shortly after I came to nanny for him, I began to pay attention to exactly what he was eating. His favorite foods, other than toast, were easy to pinpoint because he only ate a few of them: macaroni and cheese, spaghetti with meatballs, cheese quesadillas, chicken burritos, and biscuits with butter. Sometimes he also enjoyed bagels or English muffins with butter, and he would only eat a salad if it was covered in croutons (no dressing). He also enjoyed the quick breads his mother sometimes made on the weekends, especially the pumpkin and banana breads.

I saw a pattern, as I'm sure you do: Christopher loved starch! If it was made of wheat flour, he was almost surely going to like it, sugar or not. All of his favorite foods contained wheat, and I soon began to see how much of it he was eating. Whenever I see a dietary imbalance like this—a child eating an inordinate amount of one food item, no matter what it is—a red flag always goes up and my nanny sensibility compels me to say something.

So, I spoke to his mother. I told her of my concern. At first, I could tell she was a bit defensive. She didn't want to admit her baby was overweight, but she knew. I pointed out my observations about his dietary patterns. "What if," I suggested, "we tried nothing other than to change all the white flour he eats to whole-grain flour?"

His mother agreed, as long as I would take charge, because she wasn't exactly sure how to make the switch. I hurried out to the grocery and bought 100% whole wheat bread, brown rice pasta, multigrain tortillas, and whole wheat pastry flour. For good measure, I bought a package of 100% whole wheat English muffins.

The next week, I made Christopher his toast, his spaghetti with meatballs, his chicken burritos, even his biscuits, but nothing contained white flour. At first, he asked me what was "wrong" with his toast, but I assured him we were trying a more nutritious kind of bread, and being a smart boy, he agreed that this sounded like a fine idea. It still tasted pretty good, with all the butter, he admitted. I was careful not to change anything else about his favorite foods other than the whole-grain aspect, because I didn't want to change too much at once.

As the week went on, I noticed that Christopher was eating less. Two pieces of toast were enough. He didn't need four. He had one (large) helping of spaghetti, instead of two. And although he said he really liked the chicken burrito, he didn't quite finish it.

I was only with Christopher for a few months, but as I watched him grow and approach adolescence, I also watched him slim down, slowly but surely. He also seemed to have more energy, and the last I heard, he was planning to join the junior high's cross-country team. I couldn't have been more proud.

Whole-Grain Families

We eat a lot of wheat. And if you think *you* eat a lot of wheat, consider what your kids are eating. Sandwiches, tortillas, macaroni, cereal, hamburger and hot dog buns, cookies, snack cakes, biscuits, dinner rolls, spaghetti—most of the classic kid-food favorites contain a lot of wheat, mostly in the form of white flour. Wheat has a lot to recommend it. In its natural form, it contains vitamins, minerals, fiber, and plant oil, all of which can be beneficial for a child's health. We do tend to eat too much of it, throwing our diet out of balance. However, in moderation, wheat is a good food, unless your child is allergic to it or has a wheat sensitivity, or a condition such as celiac disease or even autism (see sidebar, page 73).

However, for most kids, a moderate amount of wheat is just fine. Unless we've tampered with it—which we have. What manufacturers have done in the quest to make flour last longer on the shelf without spoiling is to take out all the nutritional parts, leaving only empty starch calories. Flour contains calories, but that's about all. It's also treated with bleach so it appears snow white in color.

Enriched flour is only slightly better. Manufacturers spray vitamins and minerals back onto the starch to replace what they took out, but these chemical approximations aren't the same as the original. Mother Nature knew what she was doing when she made wheat. I'm not sure we were so wise trying to reinvent her perfect creation.

For children who struggle with being overweight or obese, white flour is a big detriment to their diet because it isn't nutrient-dense. You get a lot of calories without a lot of nutrition. Plus, like sugar, white flour is a powerful appetite stimulant. Taking apart a whole food this way confuses your body. It knows something is missing, so it keeps signaling you to eat more. It fills your children with calories but not with nutrients. This is why Christopher so often wanted another piece of toast, and then another, and another. The more white flour you eat, the more you want. Pair it up with sugar in the form of cookies and cupcakes and brownies, and you've got a perfect storm of excessive calories piled on top of appetite stimulation.

There is an old saying I've heard: "The whiter the bread, the quicker you're dead." I certainly wouldn't repeat that to a young child, but a teenager might appreciate the macabre sentiment. I think it's worth remembering privately when your child clamors for a peanut butter and jelly sandwich or a bowl of macaroni and cheese or a cookie.

How Too Much White Flour Can Affect Your Child

How bad can a slice of white bread really be? Stripped of its natural bran and germ, the sources of its fiber and nutritional content, white flour is, as far as the body and bloodstream are concerned, essentially just white sugar. In a race to shoot glucose into the bloodstream, white flour comes in a very close second to white sugar. Because they are both stripped of the natural jackets they used to wear, which break down more slowly in the body, they jolt the blood sugar into an unnaturally quick spike. As with sugar, this triggers a flood of insulin, which knocks blood sugar way back down, resulting in a ravenous hunger, just an hour or two after eating. "More toast! More cookies! More macaroni!"

Many diet plans forbid the "white foods," and they mean white flour, white sugar, white rice, and white potatoes, but at least the potatoes have some nutritional content. They come out of the earth that way. Wheat, on the other hand, is not white. (And neither are rice or sugar cane.) White flour and other processed starches are unnatural foods that provoke unnatural, extreme responses in our bodies.

Everything in the last chapter about sugar's effect on blood sugar, insulin, and behavior can also apply to white flour. Many people who are sugar sensitive are also sensitive to white flour, but not to whole wheat flour.

Another problem with white flour is what it doesn't do. White flour hardly contains any fiber compared to whole grains, and fiber is very important for children as well as adults. There are two kinds of dietary fiber: soluble and insoluble. Soluble fiber is in oats, peas, beans, apples, carrots, and citrus fruit. It helps to lower cholesterol and glucose levels when they are too high. Insoluble fiber is the rougher stuff—what they call "roughage"—that helps your child's digestive system move along more smoothly. It can help with constipation and tummy aches. It is found in whole wheat, wheat bran, and a lot of different kinds of vegetables. Eating more fruit and vegetables will add more fiber to your diet, but most kids also need the added benefit of whole grains to get enough fiber.

A little white flour now and then isn't going to hurt most healthy children. However, you may especially consider eliminating or reducing your child's consumption of white flour–based foods, such as breads and baked goods, if he or she:

- Is overweight (white flour = empty calories, but a high-fiber diet can make kids feel full longer and eat fewer calories)

> ## The Grain, the Whole Grain, and Nothing but the Grain!
>
> The ideal way to eat grains is in their whole state, even before they are broken down into flour. Whole oats, barley, brown rice, quinoa, amaranth, and bulgur wheat are all healthy, natural grains filled with fiber and minerals. The ideal way to eat grains is to steam or boil the grains in their whole form and eat them, oatmeal style.

- Seems unusually moody (white flour can cause blood sugar spikes and drops)
- Has tantrums or other behavior problems within about four hours of a meal with a lot of white flour (could also be due to unstable blood sugar)
- Is sugar sensitive (see the previous chapter)
- Is constipated or has frequent tummy aches (a possible sign of insufficient fiber intake, although check with your doctor about recurrent stomach pain)
- Gets frequent colds and other illnesses (like sugar, too much white flour could suppress immune function)

How to Make the Switch to Whole Grains

When you get used to the taste of whole-grain products, you'll begin to prefer them. But once again, take it easy. Remember the three-step approach from Chapter 2? Use it up, upgrade it, phase it out. Use up your white flour and other processed-grain products first. Then, as different things run out, such as bread or cereal or pasta or pancake mix, upgrade to a whole-grain version. For baking, first switch to unbleached flour, then try whole wheat pastry flour, which has a lighter texture than regular whole wheat flour but is much more nutritious than white flour. If you like to bake, you might even experiment with other whole-grain flours such as oat flour, corn flour, spelt flour, and flours made from non-grains such as soy and nuts. There are many delicious whole-grain breads and cereals that don't taste grainy or unpleasant at all. Eventually, you can phase white flour out of your household completely.

Many easy, quick packaged foods available now use whole grains. You can upgrade to whole grains as you are upgrading your packaged food choices. Some surprises I've found on the grocery store shelves: boxed whole-grain macaroni and cheese, instant brown rice, and quinoa pasta. For an extra-choosy child, try making both versions for a while, and mixing a little white macaroni, rice, or spaghetti with a little of the whole-grain stuff. Your more adventurous child may find that instant brown rice with a little smidge of butter is just about the same as white rice, and organic whole-grain macaroni and cheese is just as good as the stuff in the blue box. If even this is hard, begin with bread. You can buy bread made with part whole wheat flour and part white flour. It's a gateway bread! When your child gets used to the bread's being a little bit different in shade, then move to the next step. I understand some children are more sensitive to food changes than are others, but be persistent. Sometimes, children need to try things multiple times before they accept them. Then one day, out of the blue, they are munching away on their whole wheat toast with no-added-sugar jam

Sprouted

Sprouted-grain bread is a delicious, chewy, grainy treat, and even better for your body than whole-grain bread. The grains are sprouted first, meaning they are allowed to germinate, essentially turning them from grains into vegetables. The sprouted grains are then ground up and baked into loaves of bread. The most popular brand of sprouted grain bread is Food for Life. They make Ezekiel bread, as well as Ezekiel English muffins, tortillas, pasta, and cereal.

If you are used to the white stuff, the change to sprouted grains is a big step, and not everybody likes the texture. Some people love it, but how will you know if you never try? If you are stepping up your grain consumption gradually, sprouted is where you want to land.

and they are perfectly happy about it. Then you'll know you're finally on your way to whole-grain heaven.

Finally Flour-Free?

Many will be very happy replacing white flour with whole-grain flour in their family's diet, but if you want to go all the way with this, you can move toward phasing out flour-based products altogether. This may not work if you and your children really love bread and pasta. However, even reducing flour-based products can make a big difference in how you feel.

How do you do it? Keep it simple. Kids like simple food, and simple food is easy and quick to cook. I like to make whole-grain oatmeal for breakfast; brown rice with raisins and sliced almonds for lunch; and try more exotic grains for dinner, such as bulgur wheat in salads, quinoa pilaf, or millet porridge. Polenta made from whole-grain ground corn is also yummy sliced and fried in olive oil and topped with marinara sauce. There are so many delicious options, and no pressure! If your child really wants pasta, have whole-grain pasta for dinner. You don't have to phase out flour products entirely, not at all. Just open your mind to the many amazing whole-grain options available to you, and start expanding your horizons. The more varied your child's diet, the more likely he'll get the widest possible range of vitamins, minerals, and phytonutrients, the ingredients in plant foods that help us stay healthy.

Once you embrace the concept of whole grains, you and your child will begin to feel calmer and more in control because the natural rises and falls in blood sugar will become more even and less dramatic. You'll probably notice fewer digestive problems, and you might even notice a drop in your cholesterol if you are eating whole grains, too (and I hope you are!). I can almost guarantee that kids who are overweight will begin to lose weight and have less of an overactive appetite without white flour products in their diet, especially if you are also greatly reducing their processed sugar intake. Your child's body will finally understand what he is eating and can normalize its own blood sugar and weight, so his natural energy, strength, and personality can finally shine through.

About Gluten, Celiac Disease, and Autism

In addition to its dearth of nutrition, white flour has an added detriment for some children, just because it is made of wheat. Some children are allergic to wheat. Others have celiac disease, and the gluten (a complex of wheat proteins) in wheat causes an autoimmune response in their bodies, resulting in a range of dangerous symptoms, including severe gastrointestinal distress, inability to absorb nutrients, and even emotional problems. There is a group of people who also believe that some autistic children are actually intolerant of gluten and, some say, casein (a protein in dairy products).

It has become fashionable lately to give up gluten, but I don't believe this is necessary for children unless they have a sensitivity to it. However, for those who do, a life free of wheat and all other grains that contain gluten (barley, rye, spelt, and most oats, as well as some food additives) is a necessity.

It is beyond the scope of this book to go into how to do that, but if you suspect your child could have celiac disease, please talk to your doctor and check out the American Celiac Disease Alliance (http://americanceliac.org) for a lot of good information and links. You might also read my co-author Eve's book, *The Complete Idiot's Guide to Gluten-Free Eating*, for more information. There are many other good books on the subject, too.

If you have an autistic child, you should also know that, according to the World Health Organization, autism affected about 1 in 10,000 kids in 1970. Today, that number has risen to 1 in 110 children, according to the Centers for Disease Control and Prevention. Mamas, that is deeply disturbing—1 in 110 children! Although the link between autism and gluten intolerance hasn't been proved, there is a growing group of parents who say they have seen great improvements in their autistic children's communication skills with a gluten-free, casein-free diet.

If your child has been diagnosed with autism, or is showing early signs and your doctor is suggesting early intervention (because in some children, targeted behavior intervention can actually head off the disease or make it less severe, and that's exciting, too), I sincerely urge you to talk to your doctor about trying a gluten-free and casein-free diet for your child.

For more information, visit the GFCF Diet Intervention–Autism Diet Web site at www.gfcfdiet.com. Also check out the great book *Gluten-Free Kids: Raising Happy, Healthy Children with Celiac Disease, Autism, and Other Conditions* by Danna Korn.

Organic Nanny To-Do List

☐ Upgrade to bread that contains a greater percentage of whole grains than is in the bread you currently use.

☐ Try whole-grain pancakes—they are heartier and nuttier than the white-flour kind. Add a few spoonfuls of whole-grain oatmeal and some wheat germ or oat bran to the batter, for an extra nutritional boost.

☐ Experiment with different brands of whole-grain pasta, including macaroni and cheese products. Try pasta made from brown rice, quinoa, or whole wheat.

☐ Try baking with whole wheat pastry flour. Try recipes with half white flour and half whole wheat pastry flour at first, or just jump in and go for it.

☐ Try instant brown rice—as quick as instant white, but a definite upgrade. Or, invest in a rice cooker so you can make whole-grain brown rice the old-fashioned way, for maximum nutritional impact.

CHAPTER FIVE

Step 4

Ditch Dairy and
Change Your Life

I'll never forget Morty, a chubby toddler with a protruding belly who loved to tell me, "I'm the boss, and I will destroy you!" then burst into giggles. He was a Mini-Me version of his dad, a high-powered movie producer. Morty's mother was a television actress. They were all white-blond with pale skin and bright blue eyes. They looked like they were straight off the cover of *InStyle* magazine, but soon after I started caring for Morty, I became concerned.

This little guy had dark circles under his eyes, made all the more dramatic by his pale skin. He suffered from chronic diarrhea and recurrent respiratory infections, and he just didn't look healthy. It was clear something was wrong, but nobody could figure out why. His parents spent thousands of dollars on tests and medications. Then one day, it occurred to me—Morty always seemed to get sick after eating. What was he eating? His mother often gave him a glass of milk when he was hungry, and he had milk with every meal. Could it be the milk?

I told his mother my suspicion, and mainly because she was so tired of trying things that didn't work, she agreed to try eliminating milk from his diet. Bingo, at last! Once he was on a dairy-free diet, Morty's health

turned around completely. The diarrhea was resolved, his skin bright-
ened, he smiled more, and the dark circles under his eyes slowly faded.
Morty grew to love his Secret Agent Smoothies (made with almond milk,
protein powder, and blueberries, page 228) and I grew to love Morty. I
still have his picture on my dresser and his words in my memory: "Thank
you, Nanny, for taking care of my tummy!"

But What Could Possibly Be Wrong with Milk?

The notion that milk isn't good for kids shocks people because we have
been so ingrained to believe that milk is important for health—that it
"does a body good." I'm not the only one who disagrees that this is true.
For example, Walter C. Willett, MD, a professor of epidemiology and
chairman of nutrition for the Department of Nutrition at Harvard School
of Public Health wrote: "Dairy products shouldn't occupy the prominent
place they do in the U.S. Department of Agriculture food pyramid . . . Instead, the evidence shows that dietary calcium should come from a variety of sources . . . Consider dairy products as an optional part of a healthy
diet and have them in moderation, if at all."

In 1998, parenting guru Dr. Benjamin Spock, author of the world-
famous *Baby and Child Care*, amended his book to read: "Cow's milk is
not recommended for a child when he is sick—or when he is well, for
that matter. Dairy products may cause more mucus complications and
cause more discomfort with upper respiratory infections." Some thought
he was too radical. Many others, doctors and parents alike, were relieved
to have their suspicions validated by a doctor of his caliber.

Dr. Willett and Dr. Spock aren't the only doctors who believe cow's
milk is, at best, an unnatural food for children, and at worst, toxic. However, it's a logical conclusion. Milk is made for human babies and it comes
from human mothers. Cow's milk comes from cows and is made for baby
cows. It's designed to grow them to a huge size very quickly. It contains
proteins designed for a baby cow's system, not a human's.

Millions of humans all over the world cannot digest the protein in
cow's milk. Maybe your child can, but after weaning, milk has done its

job—grown a baby mammal to the point where he or she can eat solid food. Why keep feeding it to your child? After weaning, milk has served its purpose.

For years, I have been studying the effects of dairy on the human body. Much of what I've read applies to adults. For instance, dairy consumption has been closely linked to increased rates of prostate cancer in men, and the Iowa Women's Health Study suggests that women who consume more than one glass of milk per day have a 73 percent greater chance of developing ovarian cancer than do women who drink less than one glass of milk per day.

In his study of how protein turns on cancer genes, Dr. T. Colin Campbell, author of the widely acclaimed book *The China Study*, discovered that casein was the one protein that consistently promoted cancer cell growth. Casein is the dominant protein in cow's milk. In his book, Dr. Campbell lists many studies and research in which he participated that demonstrated the potential health hazards of dairy products, particularly their protein. He notes that animal protein in general seems to have a cancer-promoting effect, while protein from wheat and soy does not seem to have this same effect.

But it isn't just the protein in milk that causes trouble for health, especially in children. Several studies demonstrate that the milk sugar in dairy products could increase the risk of diabetes in children. Also, some children have a milk allergy, which is different than lactose intolerance. Within minutes or up to a few hours after consuming milk, they may have vomiting, wheezing, hives, or even go into shock.

Most children aren't actually allergic to milk, but aside from these dramatic chronic diseases, the simple fact is that most of the world's population can't digest milk once they are weaned. Nursing infants have an enzyme that breaks down the lactose in milk, but most people lose this enzyme once they stop nursing. With the exception of people who tend to be of Northern European descent, milk just isn't an appropriate food. If you drink milk or eat cheese or have an ice-cream cone and you can't digest lactose very well, you will suffer from painful gastrointestinal distress. I see this in children all the time.

I remember one little boy named Tyler who was just two years old. He didn't talk very well, but he would toddle over to the couch or the chair and press his belly into the arm or the cushion. His parents never knew what he was doing until they discovered, at a doctor's visit, that he was lactose intolerant. He was pushing his stomach against these surfaces to help relieve his pain. When they put him on a dairy-free diet, he stopped this strange behavior and became a much happier little boy.

Finally, cheese may actually be addictive. According to clinical researcher and founder and president of the Physicians Committee for Responsible Medicine, Dr. Neal Barnard has written that cheese contains a morphinelike substance produced in the cow's liver. When we eat cheese, the body breaks down this substance and releases it into our bodies, and we feel a mild opiate-like effect. Even more pronounced is the effect of casomorphins, which are opiates produced when the body breaks down casein. Dr. Barnard theorizes that cheese is actually addictive, like a drug. It makes you feel great, sure. But it's not a natural way to feel. Some scientists also theorize that this opiate-like effect is one of the reasons why nursing calms babies, and perhaps this is part of milk's design. However, once we are no longer nursing, this "high" isn't productive. We can't handle it. We have to have it, and so we eat too much cheese, with all its fat and calories.

In my own experience as a nanny, I've seen so many children begin to blossom and thrive once they got off dairy products. I've seen many families lose weight—parents and children—and achieve balance in their bodies once they kick the dairy habit, and cheese may be a big part of the reason why. Not every child reacts poorly to dairy products. Some do fine, especially if dairy is more of an occasional indulgence, like a bowl of macaroni and cheese or a small ice cream cone every so often (as opposed to every day). However, for other children like Morty, dairy products are best left behind.

You probably grew up with milk on your cereal, cheese on your hamburger, and ice cream after dinner, and you think you can't live without butter. I understand the power of habit and tradition. However, there are compelling reasons to consider that neither you nor your children should be swilling the milk and piling on the cheese.

My personal experience with giving up dairy products has been wonderful. When I decided to ditch dairy for good, my skin got more radiant, my face got clearer, and much to my relief, I don't crave dairy at all. Not even cheese!

Not only is it easier on your body not to have to try to digest cow's milk, but if you don't eat dairy, you and your children will probably consume less fat and fewer calories. For kids struggling with weight issues, this is a big plus. Many fatty, creamy sauces and dressings contain milk or cream or butter or all of the above. The same goes for rich, fattening desserts.

Many people who give up dairy find that if they decide to try it again, they react with major allergy symptoms.

How Too Much Dairy Can Affect Your Child

You may especially consider eliminating or reducing your child's consumption of dairy-containing foods, such as milk, cheese, cottage cheese, ice cream, and yogurt made with cow's milk, if he or she has any of the following health or behavioral issues:

- *A weight problem.* Dairy products can add a lot of fat and calories to a child's diet, compared to fruit, vegetables, and whole grains.
- *Digestive issues.* Many children have problems digesting lactose. Lactose intolerance affects about 95 percent of Asian Americans, 74 percent of Native Americans, 70 percent of African Americans, 53 percent of Mexican Americans, and 15 percent of Caucasians.
- *Respiratory or congestion issues.* Dairy appears to increase congestion and mucus in the body. One of the first things people often say they notice when they give up dairy products is a noticeable clearing of congestion and easier breathing.
- *Food allergies.* If a child is sensitive to foods, milk may be one of them, and it's in many processed foods, so read the labels.
- *Iron deficiency.* The calcium in dairy foods can inhibit iron absorption.

Milk and Health Conditions

In his exhaustive research on the effects of dairy products, Dr. Robert M. Kradjian, a former chief of general surgery, found published studies and reports linking every single one of the following conditions to the human consumption of dairy products:

Allergies
Anemia
Arthritis
Asthma
Bedwetting
Cancer
Childhood diabetes
Colic
Contamination of milk with blood and white (pus) cells
Contamination of milk with chemicals and insecticides
Ear and tonsil infections
Heart disease
Infections, such as salmonella
Intestinal bleeding
Intestinal irritation
Leukemia
Lymphoma
Sinusitis

After his discovery, he penned a famous letter to his patients, urging them not to consume dairy products. In the letter, often called the "Milk Letter" (you can see the whole thing at www.notmilk.com/kradjian.html), he wrote: "Don't drink milk for health. I am convinced on the weight of scientific evidence that it does not 'do a body good.' Inclusion of milk will only reduce your diet's nutritional value and safety. Most of the people on this planet live very healthfully without cow's milk. You can, too."

- *Juvenile arthritis.* According to an article in a 1985 issue of the *Journal of the Royal Society of Medicine*, an eight-year-old girl with a mysterious case of juvenile rheumatoid arthritis had a complete remission of symptoms when she stopped drinking milk.
- *Autism.* Although the link between gluten (protein in wheat), casein (a protein in milk), and autism is as yet unproven, many people strongly believe that autistic children have a metabolic disorder that causes casein to have an opiate-like effect on them even more pronounced than it may have in people without the disorder. Many parents say that taking their autistic children off all gluten and casein has resulted in dramatic improvement in behavior and responsiveness. For more information and resources about this issue, see the sidebar about autism in the previous chapter.

Milk Step-Down

People worry that if they take milk away from their children, they won't get enough calcium. However, many vegetables and other foods contain calcium, and calcium is also added to many nondairy milks in the same proportion it occurs in regular milk. Add plenty of calcium-rich plant foods, and your child will have all the calcium she needs! Calcium-rich choices include:

- Dark leafy greens
- Broccoli
- Kidney beans
- Chickpeas (and hummus)
- Green beans
- Almonds and almond butter
- Sesame seeds and sesame butter (also called tahini)
- Even pasta and bread

As with the other food items you have decided to phase out of your life, you can phase out dairy gradually. Or, if you really think your child is having a serious problem with dairy products and you want to get rid of them, just do it. Pour the milk down the sink. Switching to nondairy milk is so easy because there are many delicious nondairy milks available now that appeal to kids. Try soy milk, almond milk, coconut milk, rice milk, hemp milk, hazelnut milk, or oat milk.

For some families, cheese is harder (although some children don't like cheese, in which case it's a nonissue). It might be that opiate effect I mentioned earlier in this chapter, or just habit, but whatever it is, some people find it extremely difficult to give up cheese.

The good news is that once you haven't had cheese for a while, you start to crave it less often. First, upgrade by experimenting with dairy-free cheeses. Those that are truly dairy free will be marked "vegan." (Some others that say they are dairy-free contain casein.) Some vegan brands I like are Follow Your Heart, Daiya, and Teese. You may not be a fan of dairy-free cheeses. They don't taste exactly like regular cheese, and you may get used to them, or not. You can always just leave the cheese off what you are eating, to let the other flavors shine through. Cheese tends to dominate any dish. Can you have a sandwich without the cheese? Do you have to add cheese to your corn chips, or can you just dip them in salsa or hummus? I highly recommend cheese-free pizza. All the fun and a fraction of the fat and calories! Almost any pizza delivery place will leave off the cheese if you request it.

Another dairy product popular with children is yogurt. However, you don't need to give up yogurt. There are some excellent dairy-free yogurts in delicious flavors, including those made with soy milk, coconut milk, and almond milk. Again, however, check the label—at least one popular brand of soy yogurt contains some dairy.

So many people in recent years have gone dairy-free that it's easier than ever before. With a few healthful replacements, you may find nobody misses dairy at all. If your last holdout is cream in your coffee, Mama, I suggest trying Silk Creamer, in plain, French vanilla, or hazelnut. Yum. It doesn't taste exactly like milk, and it does contain some sugar, but it's a taste that many people grow to love, and a cup of good Cuban coffee with a little Silk Creamer is a relatively healthful indulgence for a mama who needs to get through the morning!

Cows Are Mamas, Too!

I am a strong proponent of a dairy-free diet for children, for health reasons. However, there are other deeply compelling reasons to ditch the white stuff. Cows must be continually artificially inseminated so they are pregnant as often as possible, so that they can give birth and produce milk. A cow that hasn't just given birth won't produce milk. Why would she? Already, we are messing with nature, forcing the cows to become pregnant. But then, it gets worse.

When a cow gives birth to a baby cow, she is added to the dairy herd. When she gives birth to a male, the baby calf is taken away from her, often just minutes after birth. If you've ever seen a video of a mama cow bellowing for her baby, who is being tossed onto a truck to be sold for cheap veal, I bet you will never want to buy industrial dairy products again.

Plus, because of the constant milking, many dairy cows have chronic breast infections, which means the milk contains pus and blood cells. I would never want any of the children in my care to drink up their milk. Dairy milk does not make for a peaceful meal. Lactating cows are mamas, too, even if they aren't human. Stand together, mamas of all species! A mother's milk is for her own baby, not for adults of some other species.

I suggest a dairy-free experiment for your family. Give it up for one month, and see what happens. I know so many happy, healthy, strong, energetic, beautiful children who never touch a glass of milk or a slice of "processed cheese food." Maybe your family is fine with dairy products, but why not see if things get better without them? If you try it, I'm betting you're going to witness something akin to a miracle.

Giving up dairy can trigger beautiful changes in your children, who will not only start to develop a sense of pride in eating the way you do, but also a sense of compassion for everyone on Earth—humans, animals, the Earth itself. This is how you begin to build a reverence for life into your family's very fabric. It's a way to pass along not just good health habits but good values, too.

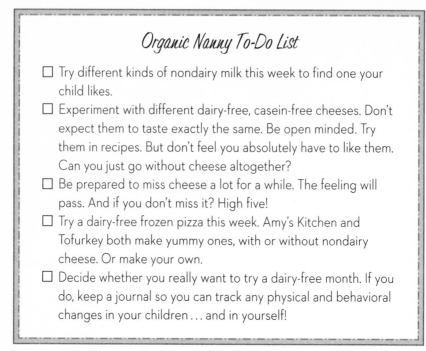

Organic Nanny To-Do List

☐ Try different kinds of nondairy milk this week to find one your child likes.

☐ Experiment with different dairy-free, casein-free cheeses. Don't expect them to taste exactly the same. Be open minded. Try them in recipes. But don't feel you absolutely have to like them. Can you just go without cheese altogether?

☐ Be prepared to miss cheese a lot for a while. The feeling will pass. And if you don't miss it? High five!

☐ Try a dairy-free frozen pizza this week. Amy's Kitchen and Tofurkey both make yummy ones, with or without nondairy cheese. Or make your own.

☐ Decide whether you really want to try a dairy-free month. If you do, keep a journal so you can track any physical and behavioral changes in your children . . . and in yourself!

CHAPTER SIX

Step 5

Eat More Veggies, Less Meat, and with L.O.V.E.

Animals are my friends and I don't eat my friends.
—George Bernard Shaw

*T*he California sun illuminated the cottage and garden as I pulled into the drive. The Pacific Ocean in the distance sparkled and I had an immediate feeling of calm and well-being, before I even met my newest clients—a novelist, his holistic healer wife, and their family of four gorgeous children, Matthew, Sam, Raina, and Bella. As they all came out to the garden to meet me, I felt so welcome, and I felt such radiating health and energy from all of them. I would soon realize how much they had to teach me.

The children, ages two, seven, fourteen, and sixteen, were the picture of glowing health. As I came to know and love them, I learned that this family ate no processed foods, no meat, and no dairy products. They ate fresh, whole foods from their own garden and from the farmers' market, and nobody complained. In fact, the children loved to eat real, fresh food, and they loved to help prepare it, too. The kitchen was always full of children, grabbing fruit, helping to assemble salads, or (not the little ones) chopping vegetables. Until that time, I'd never seen anything like it. These children rarely got sick, never had ear infections, and had never needed antibiotics. They were living the Organic Nanny dream.

I was fascinated by this family because I could see all the principles I've always preached playing themselves out in the real world, confirming everything I'd always believed. This was the first family I'd ever cared for that was not riddled with arguments, stress, and fighting. The children were talented and involved in the arts, and their parents cultivated and encouraged their children's natural creativity. They also cultivated and encouraged an appreciation for the natural world, and a deep reverence for all life. I'm sure that a lot of this came out of how they were raised, in addition to what they were eating. They had the whole package, and they were a beautiful model for the family that wants to live a more natural, harmonized life.

I think what struck me the most about this family was how drastically it contradicted the stereotype of the vegan family. These children weren't pale, or underweight, or sickly, or weak . They were strong and healthy and intelligent. The food they ate was so beautiful, so full of life energy, that eating animal products had become simply irrelevant to them. I remember wishing I could hold them up as an example to the whole world, to shout, "Look, everyone! Look what children can be when you start feeding them more nutritious food!"

Perhaps I'm being dramatic. (Remember, it's the Cuban in me.) However, I sincerely and passionately believe in my Organic Nanny heart that what this family illustrates can be a reality for any family. I believe that no child ever needs to eat animals, and while many children can eat meat and do fine, it's certainly not necessary for health. I also believe that the best thing you can do for your children's diet is to make fruit and vegetables the centerpiece of the meal.

The Wonderful World of Plant Foods

Think for a moment about sweet, juicy fruit. Crisp apples, tender pears, juicy grapes, candy-sweet blueberries, tangy strawberries, fun-to-peel clementines, rich bananas, succulent peaches and plums, wedges of watermelon in the summer, warm apples and cinnamon in the winter . . . fruit is such a luxurious, beautiful food group. Why don't our children eat more of it?

Now think about vegetables. Sweet crunchy carrots, savory green beans with crispy onions, crunchy lettuce, sweet potatoes with maple syrup, snappy bell pepper strips dipped in hummus, tender sweet corn, crispy baked kale chips, summer squashes sautéed in butter, juicy tomatoes (I know, they are actually a fruit, but bear with me) . . . vegetables are densely packed with nutrients and offer such a broad variety of tastes. Why don't our children eat more of them?

But I understand how hard it can be. The family I mention at the beginning of this chapter had it easy in some ways. The parents were vegetarians and they had raised their children that way. They also had plenty of money to buy the very best organic produce, they lived in a place where they could get a lot of amazing local food, and they could also afford a personal chef. Most of us don't have those luxuries.

However, I have devised a system that can help families move from where they are now to a more natural diet that is passionately focused on plant foods and less on animal products. I introduced you to this concept in the first chapter, but now I'm going to show you how to make it work, to phase out the meat and phase in the plant kingdom. I call it eating with L.O.V.E.

As you may remember, L.O.V.E. is a system that can help to guide your dietary choices in the right direction. It's an acronym that stands for what, ideally, your meals should be made of. *L* stands for Local, as in local produce and other locally produced food items. *O* stands for Organic, as in, as much of the food you eat as possible should be free of pesticides and other chemicals. *V* stands for vegetable-centric, vegetarian, or vegan. You can take this step as far as you like. I'll show you how. Finally, *E* stands for Environmental. When you eat with the Earth's well-being in mind, you proactively help to preserve the environment for your children's future.

You won't always be able to eat every meal according to all of these principles, but this is just a place to start. Keep it in your mind when you shop, when you cook, and when you sit down at the table with your children. Talk about it, so they know what it means, too. Discuss the importance of each of the steps, and show them through your actions that you care about the quality and content of their food and yours. Let L.O.V.E. work its magic on your family, and witness the calm and loving influence it can have.

L Is for Local

Let's begin where you live. The first part of L.O.V.E. is about eating food produced right nearby. Why does that matter?

Eating local food matters in many ways. First of all, buying it involves you in your community. You are financially supporting local food producers, rather than sending your money far away. This can give you a comforting sense of support. When you support your community, it will support you. A community is like a family, and knowing you are part of it can be a great thing for your physical as well as mental health. It will give your children a sense of belonging, stability, roots. It will also nurture in your children a sense of responsibility for others, rather than selfishness. Spend your money locally, and you nurture your community right back.

Eating local food also helps you get more in tune with the natural as well as the social world around you. You become aware of the influence of the weather and the seasons on local food production. You begin to eat more in sync with the Earth's rhythm, and that feels good. I also believe it can make you healthier.

Local food also just tastes better. It hasn't been coated with wax or picked early and gassed to ripeness, because it doesn't have to survive a long journey from wherever to you. Often, local food was picked the day you eat it, or just a few days before, rather than weeks before. It has a more ephemeral quality, too. It may not last long, but at its peak, it's something very special. You know what I mean if you've ever picked and eaten berries or apples at a local farm, or had sweet corn plucked from the stalk on the same day, before the natural sugars turn to starch, or if you've bought warm peaches from a roadside stand or grapes off a vine, or plucked a pea pod and eaten the peas right out of the shell.

Be a Locavore

Fortunately, eating local food has become something of a fad, but my hope is that it will catch on so strongly that it will become a new way of thinking. People who practice local eating and buying call themselves locavores, and my heart warms when I see the bumper stickers and T-shirts proudly proclaiming locavore status, or encouraging others to "Think globally, eat locally!" Recently, I saw T-shirts made for babies that said, "Locally grown." I love that! Every child should be locally grown, in more than just the literal sense. All children should be an integral part of the community, nourished physically and emotionally by their immediate environment.

Another benefit of local food is its nutritional value. The time between harvesting and consuming matters. The longer a vegetable or fruit sits before you eat it, the more nutritional value it loses. It gets older and less fresh. Produce sitting on a truck traveling halfway across the country or even the planet simply won't be as fresh and vibrant and nutritious as produce picked the day you eat it. (And just think of all the fossil fuel expended to get that produce to you—not good for the planet, either.)

Local food also tends to be a real bargain. All that time and shipping adds to the cost of nonlocal food, and because it is seasonal, it also tends to be less expensive than a nonlocal product bought out of season (such as those mealy, tasteless tomatoes in the winter).

Local food is often organic, but even when it's not, the small farmers who sell their wares at the farmers' market often don't need to use much in the way of chemicals, because they aren't mass producing and they aren't shipping. Sometimes, the farmers can't afford to be certified organic, but they will tell you that they really are organic. In any case, the beauty of buying from a local farmer is that you can ask about pesticide use. And if you grow food yourself, in your own backyard, well . . . you can't get much more local than that.

Where do you find local produce? In the summer, it's easy, and in some parts of the country, it's always easy. More cold-weather climates are opening winter farmers' markets, too, although their offerings will be different than in the summer, of course. Farmers' markets are always seasonal, so winter markets may offer more winter squashes, winter greens, and also animal products such as meat and cheese.

Not every community has an abundance of local products. You might live in a place that is hundreds of miles from any farm. Or, maybe you just aren't aware of the hidden jewels in or just outside your community. However, most cities have farmers' markets these days, and organic farmers will be there, selling what they grow. They may be doing the traveling to get to you. Also, many supermarkets now label their local products, in response to the locavore trend.

Not all local food is plant food, but in general, it tends to be mostly fruit and vegetables, and sometimes dairy products. Some places also sell local meat raised on small family farms. This can be a great transition from feedlot beef and other factory-farmed meat and poultry. Local meat is an *upgrade*.

Eating local food is so rewarding, and a great way to involve your children in food selection. I hope you'll give it a try this week. Also consider that the *L* in L.O.V.E. can apply to more than food. Bring your children to local festivals, street fairs, outdoor concerts, and parks. Instead of staying in and watching television, consider taking a walk, chatting with the neighbors, or going downtown and people-watching.

This is all part of living a more local life. Children have a lot of energy and they need fresh air and sunshine and interaction with people. Give them room to run and play, even as they get older. Take your preteens to a park with a jungle gym and swings and big open spaces, and stand back. Just watch what happens. When you really live in the present moment, right there where you are, instead of through a smartphone or a video game or a television show, life becomes more vivid and real, and you remember how to interact with people who are actually standing there in front of you. To me, this is all part of local, and should definitely be a part of life.

O Is for Organic

The next word in your L.O.V.E. mantra is absolutely essential to the health and well-being of your family. It is Organic. You probably already

What Is a CSA?

"CSA" stands for Community Supported Agriculture, and it represents an exciting movement in local living. If your community has a CSA, you can sign up with a local farmer, pay a set price at the beginning of the growing season, and then receive a box of fresh vegetables, often picked that very morning, from the farmer, about once a week. You might pick up the box at the farm, or at a local farmers' market or other pickup location.

Everything you receive will be seasonal, local, and adapted for your own climate. Every week, you'll get something different, according to what is ready for harvest. In spring, you might get fresh greens such as baby lettuces, kale, collard greens, and green onions. In the summer, prepare for a bounty of tomatoes and peppers, onions and garlic, potatoes and corn, summer squash and zucchini, and whatever else the farmer has planted that year.

In the fall, your box may be filled with winter squashes such as butternut and pumpkin, a new crop of sweet greens such as collards and chard, and other produce that stores well, such as more onions, garlic, and cabbages. Some CSAs also have fruit, from strawberries to apples, and some offer shares of freshly baked bread, eggs from their own chickens, even bouquets of flowers.

When you pick up your box, you can chat with the farmer and learn about the current growing season and how the crops are doing. It will give you a fresh perspective on your salad, and you can also feel good about supporting your local farmer and community by buying food grown not far from where you live. It's a beautiful deal, and many smaller families will go in on a share together so nothing is wasted.

Ask at your local farmers' market, food co-op, or just ask your healthiest friends if your community has a CSA. Or, look for one on the Local Harvest Web site: www.localharvest.org. It lists hundreds of CSAs and other sources for fresh local food in its searchable database.

suspect that this word is important to me, considering I call myself the Organic Nanny, but I have a very good reason: organic food is free from chemicals, and I believe the fewer chemicals children ingest, the healthier they will be.

You probably don't need me to prove to you that chemicals are harmful for children. However, the research is out there. Some of the more obvious exposure dangers have to do with children who live in rural areas or whose parents are actual farmworkers. For example, pregnant women who actually work with pesticides, or who live in areas that are heavily sprayed, were more likely to give birth to children with birth defects such as cleft palates or limb defects. Many pesticides are also neurotoxins with demonstrated effects on learning ability, IQ, and behavior in mammals. In one study of children living in the Yaqui Valley in Sonora, Mexico, an area of high pesticide use, comparing them to children living in the foothills with little pesticide exposure, the children in the valley scored worse on tests of memory, eye-hand coordination, drawing skill, and stamina than did children in the foothills.

But what about when children eat nonorganic foods? The exposure to pesticides is certainly less dramatic than if the children were to inhale pesticides or be around them daily. However, the USDA says significantly more pesticides residues are on conventional produce than on organic produce. Conventional produce doesn't usually exceed government-set standards, but why take a chance with even a little pesticide? Organic produce is simply purer and safer, even if most studies show that the nutritional content is about the same in organic and conventional produce.

Some people object to organic food because it is more expensive, and they aren't sure it really makes any difference. This is certainly a legitimate concern, and if you can't afford organic produce, then I urge you to wash your produce very well. However, some of the pesticide soaks into the produce and can't be washed off, so I always encourage parents to buy organic produce *whenever they can.* If you have the option and the resources, then why not limit your children's pesticide exposure in every possible way? It just makes good sense.

Fortunately, there are inexpensive ways to go organic:

- Buy from local farmers who don't use chemicals, even if they aren't officially certified organic.

- Look for sales at your local natural foods market or the health food aisle of your grocery store. When organic canned tomatoes go on sale, stock up. When organic apples go on sale, eat lots of apples that week.
- Shop around. Some places charge more for organic food than do others. Even Super Walmart is getting into the organic game and offering organic food at just a little bit more than conventional food. If Walmart is your best option to afford organic food for your children, then go for it.
- Go online. I'm beginning to see more packaged organic products available for great prices online. For example, I recently saw Sesame Street Organic Juice Boxes at Amazon.com—forty juice boxes for just over twenty dollars! Who would have guessed? Hooray for Sesame Street and its organic campaign! Even Elmo is going organic!
- Grow your own. Plant a small organic garden in your yard, or just grow a few vegetables in pots out on a small porch or window box. Let your kids help. Kids love to plant gardens and watch them grow.

Organic produce has other advantages, too. It cannot contain food additives such as preservatives, flavor enhancers, and artificial colors and flavors. It is also better for the environment because organic farming doesn't use any chemical pesticides and fertilizers, and organic farming methods specifically reduce pollution and conserve natural resources. Organic farming is less wasteful and less toxic.

I get that there are problems with the organic movement. It isn't perfect, and not every organic food producer always follows the rules. However, it is definitely a step in the right direction, especially for children.

"Organic" can also apply to meat and dairy products, if you eat those. Cows who give organic milk must be fed organic food and cannot be fed bovine growth hormone (rBGH), which many conventional farmers feed their dairy cows to force them to produce more milk than they normally would. (Fortunately, many companies, even nonorganic ones, are now pledging not to use bovine growth hormone. Look at the label on your milk and avoid this unnatural hormone, if you can!)

Animals slaughtered to make organic meat must also be fed organic food and supposedly treated in a more humane way than are conventional feedlot or factory-farmed animals. The same goes for chickens that lay organic eggs. Although I recommend reducing or even eliminating these animal products, going organic is a way to begin upgrading your choices as you phase them out of your diet.

And speaking of steps, let's think about how you can phase in organic produce. Let's talk about the Dirty Dozen.

The Dirty Dozen

The Dirty Dozen are the twelve foods most heavily saturated with pesticides, according to the Environmental Working Group (EWG). The Clean 15 are the foods that, even when they are not organic, tend to be pretty lightly sprayed or not sprayed at all with chemicals. As you begin your organic transition, start with the Dirty Dozen foods and switch those to organic. Don't worry about other produce items. Eventually, see if you can buy organic everything except the Clean 15. Also consider that a food with a thick skin you peel off and don't eat won't be as affected by pesticides as is a food with an edible thin skin.

Here is the Environmental Working Group's most recent list, which it updates yearly:

Dirty Dozen
1. Apples
2. Celery
3. Strawberries
4. Peaches
5. Spinach
6. Imported nectarines
7. Imported grapes
8. Sweet bell peppers
9. Potatoes
10. Domestic blueberries
11. Lettuce
12. Kale/collard greens

Clean 15

1. Onion
2. Sweet corn
3. Pineapples
4. Avocado
5. Asparagus
6. Sweet peas
7. Mangoes
8. Eggplant
9. Domestic cantaloupe
10. Kiwi
11. Cabbage
12. Watermelon
13. Sweet potatoes
14. Grapefruit
15. Mushrooms

You can check the current list on the EWG's web page at www.ewg
.org/foodnews/summary/.

Finally, the *O* in L.O.V.E. doesn't apply to just food. You can live a
more organic life in so many different ways. Your cleaning products, personal hygiene products, pet products,
linens, paint and carpeting, furniture, clothing, and even the
gifts you buy for others can
be organic or made with organic materials. There are so
many ways children can be
exposed to chemicals in their
very own homes. I say, get the chemicals out, as much as you possibly can! We
will probably never be able to live in a completely chemical-free environment. Too much pollution and contamination has built up, and even
newborn babies have residues of pesticides and other chemicals in their

Organic Voices

High-tech tomatoes. Mysterious milk.
Super squash. Are we supposed to eat
this stuff? Or is it going to eat us?

—*Anita Manning*

blood. However, you can make a big impact on chemical exposure in an easy way. Start with your food. I'll talk more about how to clean the chemicals out of your home and go organic in this important way in Chapter 8.

V Is for Vegetable-Centric, Vegetarian, or Vegan

Mother Earth knows how to feed us. She provides us with beautiful plants—luscious fruit, delicious vegetables, and . . . animals? But wait, are the animals fellow denizens of Earth, or are they just there for us to eat? Or both?

This isn't an easy question for many people to answer. As a culture, we love animals. Children, in particular, have a natural affinity for animals. Children are naturally compassionate. They delight in the natural world. When they see a dog, a cat, a bird, a pig, a cow, they laugh and point and want to touch.

Yet, we are also a culture very accustomed to eating animals. In the past fifty years, meat consumption in the United States has more than doubled. We pet dogs and cats and parakeets, and we eat cows and pigs and chickens. And sometimes we pet cows and pigs and chickens, at county fairs, as they stand in pens over signs labeling them BEEF and PORK and POULTRY.

I don't eat meat now, but I ate meat as a child. Being vegetarian was unheard of in my culture. However, we didn't eat meat at every meal, and the meat we did eat was a whole different animal, pardon the pun. A roast chicken or pig marked special occasions, not daily dinner. When we did eat meat, it was from an animal who ate grass, lived in the sun, and was freshly killed just for the meal, not to sit in a supermarket wrapped in plastic, and certainly not after a life contained in a feed lot, a battery cage, or a dark, crowded barn.

Tata would bring home a chicken and pluck the feathers herself. She would sing Cuban songs to the poor little bird, and always thanked it for giving its life so that her children and grandchildren could grow strong. Cooking a meal that included meat was a special, prolonged, celebratory process that allowed us all to look forward to the dinner as something of great value. There was a sense of reverence about food in our household and in our culture—a sense of appreciation, too. I believe it made the food taste better, and I know food so fresh and so recently plucked from the Earth filled us with vitality and energy.

The world is different now. People rarely eat meat the way we did when I was a child. Even then, I still felt bad for that poor chicken, and conflicted about the process, so it wasn't hard for me to give up meat.

It might be harder for you. Giving up meat when you are used to eating it is no easy task, but I do believe it is a worthwhile pursuit, or goal, for the health and well-being of adults and children. Certainly, we can survive on meat and dairy products, if we must, but it's not necessary, and the way our culture chooses to slaughter and process animals into meat is oftentimes cruel, inhumane, and unsanitary.

If you do choose to eat meat, there are good ways to upgrade the process. Buy local meat from small family farms that use organic practices and humane slaughtering methods. Eat it on special occasions only. And always give thanks, whether you are religious or not, for the life given up so that you can eat. I hope you will think about this.

Or you may decide you just aren't comfortable with eating meat and you would like to phase it out. I love hearing this from my clients, and I'm always ready to help. There are many ways to get inspired in your journey toward going vegetarian or vegan. Books, movies, magazines, and videos can help encourage you and offer you a sense of community. Beautiful, delicious recipes abound on the Internet, and I bet you even have a few vegetarian friends.

Many people I know who raise vegetarian children were first inspired to do so by the disturbing stories or images they encountered in books or movies, and yes, many other books for adults contain long chapters and passages on the horrors of factory farms, egg production operations, feedlots, and slaughterhouses. I'm not going to go into that here because I don't think this is appropriate for children, and because if you want to know more about these disturbing facts, you can read one of those other books or see one of the movies on this subject.

What I will tell you, however, is that there are many known health benefits to a vegetarian diet, as well as a vegan diet, not to mention those

Veg Vocabulary Lesson

Vegetarians aren't all the same, and different terms refer to different approaches. Here are some words you may have heard, and exactly what they mean:

Vegetarian: Someone who does not eat animals, including poultry, fish, and shellfish. The word is also sometimes used to mean someone who doesn't eat any animal products at all, including dairy products.

Strict vegetarian: Someone who does not eat any products from animals, including flesh, dairy products, or even honey, which is extracted from bee hives (often at the expense of the bees).

Vegan: A strict vegetarian. The term also can refer to people who do everything they can to avoid using animal products in other aspects of life, such as in their personal products (from shampoo to lipstick) and clothing (no leather, wool, or silk). This kind of vegan is also sometimes called an ethical vegan.

Lacto-vegetarian: Someone who does not eat meat, poultry, or seafood, but does eat dairy products such as milk and cheese.

Lacto-ovo-vegetarian: Someone who does not eat meat, poultry, or seafood, but does eat dairy products and eggs.

Pescatarian: Someone who does not eat meat or poultry but does eat fish (not technically a vegetarian, but some people consider this a loose form of vegetarian).

Flexitarian: A new word that refers to people who eat a vegetarian or vegan diet most of the time, but are not strict and will occasionally eat animal products. Some people are systematic about it, only eating animal products on the weekends, on holidays, or while on vacation.

Fruitarian: Someone who only eats fruit, nuts, and seeds. Some people consider themselves fruitarians if most of their diet is fruit, nuts, and seeds.

Raw foodist: Someone who never eats cooked food, or food that has been heated above 104°F. Some raw foodists are vegan, and some will include raw fish in their diet.

of a diet that is primarily composed of plant foods, even if it also includes some animal products.

For example, according to the World Health Organization, dietary factors account for at least 30 percent of all cancers in Western countries, and one of the most obvious links researchers have found is that people who avoid meat are much less likely to develop cancer. One Harvard study showed that people who eat meat every day have three times the risk of colon cancer, compared to those who rarely eat meat. Cooked meat contains a number of known carcinogenic compounds, especially when it is charred on a grill. Other studies suggest that women with higher body fat are more prone to breast cancer, because body fat produces estrogen. Meat eaters in general ten to have higher body fat than vegetarians. By contrast, people who eat the most fruit and vegetables tend to have the least cancer.

According to another study published in *The Archives of Internal Medicine* in 2009, which looked at the dietary habits of 500,000 American men and women, those who ate the most red meat and processed meat were the most likely to die at a younger age, and most often from heart disease or cancer.

Meat consumption has also been linked to obesity, osteoporosis, and dementia. But what does that have to do with children? These are largely adult diseases of aging, right?

First of all, people tend to prefer the foods they ate as children. When you feed your children, it isn't just about that meal. It's about a lifetime of eating habits becoming established *right now.* Remember the McDonald's Effect? When children associate junk food and high-fat food and other unhealthy foods with comfort, home, and *you,* then they will always prefer those foods, and someday, even if they choose to eat a healthier diet than they eat now, they will have to work very, very hard to maintain it.

On the other hand, children who grow up accustomed to eating a plant-based diet full of fruit, vegetables, and whole grains will always prefer those foods, for exactly the same reason—they associate the foods with comfort, home, and *you.* Changing your children's diet to a mostly or entirely plant-based diet is a gift that will keep on giving for the rest of their lives.

Read Aloud

One of my favorite children's books is called *That's Why We Don't Eat Animals* by Ruby Roth. This book is perfect for those parents who want extra support in their quest to raise vegan or vegetarian children. Don't read it to your children if you are still on the fence, though—or still feeding them meat. The message in this book is clear and without wiggle room, and a child who is eating meat could become upset by it. Why? Perhaps because children's hearts connect with what they already know.

Also, chronic diseases people tend to get when they are older don't just pop up out of nowhere. In many cases, these illnesses have been developing for years and years, and bad health habits that start in childhood could set up your child for a future of poor health.

Finally, you and your child can bask in the warm and fuzzy feeling you get when you embrace a cruelty-free diet. It's a beautiful reward for a lovely and healthful way to eat, and I highly recommend it for everyone. When your child pets a chicken or a pig at a farm and then goes home and eats a chicken or a pig, it can set up an internal conflict. When you don't eat the chicken or the pig (or the cow or the turkey), you don't have to try to explain to your child why it's okay to love something and then eat it.

That being said, I do recognize how hard this is, and I don't want you to feel guilty. Every family is different, and has different needs. I also believe each individual person has a diet that is right for him or her. Some people thrive on a vegan diet. Others believe they don't. All I can tell you is that *everybody* thrives on a diet rich in whole plant foods, no matter what else it might contain. The more plants you can fit into your diet, the better. See if you can encourage your entire family to become plant-consumers, and you'll all be much healthier. In fact, the American Dietetic Association wrote this, in their position statement on vegetarian diets:

It is the position of the American Dietetic Association that appropriately planned vegetarian diets, including total vegetarian or vegan diets, are healthful, nutritionally adequate, and may provide health benefits in the prevention and treatment of certain diseases. Well-planned vegetarian diets are appropriate for individuals during all stages of the life cycle, including pregnancy, lactation, infancy, childhood, and adolescence, and for athletes. . . . An evidence-based review showed that vegetarian diets can be nutritionally adequate in pregnancy and result in positive maternal and infant health outcomes. The results of an evidence-based review showed that a vegetarian diet is associated with a lower risk of death from ischemic heart disease. Vegetarians also appear to have lower low-density lipoprotein cholesterol levels, lower blood pressure, and lower rates of hypertension and type 2 diabetes than non-vegetarians. Furthermore, vegetarians tend to have a lower body mass index and lower overall cancer rates.

Obviously, of course, you can't just stop eating meat and dairy products and expect to be healthy. You also have to eat a wide variety of plant foods and be sure you have adequate intake of vitamin B_{12} and calcium. This is exactly why many families decide that a vegetarian or vegan diet won't work for their children, who won't eat very many other foods. This is exactly why I want you to focus first on a veg-centric diet. I don't want to rush you or push you out of your comfort zone. Well, maybe just a little out of your comfort zone, but not so far that you'll leap backward and give up on your entire health quest. Many children can eat only the occasional meat product and seem to do just fine. They will fit right in with their peers and grow up perfectly in line with the constructs of our current society, as it has been rolling along for the last few decades.

But as you get more comfortable with an increasingly plant-based diet, perhaps you will decide to phase out the animal products, first by upgrading them, and then by reducing them until they are only a small part of your diet. Or no part of your diet at all.

Let's also acknowledge that eating meat is an emotional subject for many people, both those who choose to do it and those who choose not to do it. You can be feeding your child the healthiest diet on the planet, and people will still tell you that you are being a bad parent, whether you

Farm Field Trip

A visit to a farm that rescues farm animals, or to an organic farm that produces vegetables and keeps animals as pets (not as food animals), can be a fun and enlightening experience for children. If you have a farm like that near you, take a day to visit (with the farmer's permission, of course). Make it a field trip. Bring an organic picnic, pet the animals, and learn about how farming was meant to be. When you see how much animals charm your child, perhaps you will be further motivated not to contribute to the creatures' slaughter.

are feeding your child a vegan diet or one that includes organic grass-fed or pasture-raised meat and poultry. This is why you absolutely have to know in your heart that you are doing the right thing for your family. It's also extremely helpful if you can find a support system of other mamas who are doing what you do, too.

But nobody is going to give you trouble for eating more vegetables. So let's talk about how to do that.

The Cult of Protein

"But where do you get your protein?" It's the number one question people ask those who abstain from animal products. The implication: "If you don't eat animals, you must be nutritionally deprived." Or worse yet: "If you don't eat animals, you are depriving your children of good nutrition."

Mamas, protein is not the answer to the question of health. In fact, too much protein can be dangerous. It's hard on the kidneys, it can contribute to dehydration, and on a perhaps shallower level, it can give you really bad breath. We all need protein, but children and adults can get all they need from plant foods, including whole grains, beans, and many vegetables. Indulge in those and save your health.

How to Go Veg-Centric, Vegetarian, or Vegan

Certainly you must know the drill by now. First, you let it run out. Then you upgrade it. Then you phase it out. For this step, you will be doing two things at once—phasing out meat and phasing *in* more vegetables and fruit.

First, you don't need to throw away all the meat in your refrigerator and freezer. Just start eating it a little less often. A lot of people like to start by trying Meatless Mondays. Meatless Mondays is a campaign that has been around since 2003, and thousands of families have adopted it. Just start with one meatless day a week, and see how it goes. See if you feel so good that you might just want to add another day.

Meanwhile, as you are using up meat, don't buy any more conventional meat. If you do feel you need to or want to have more meat, upgrade to organic meat, preferably locally raised on a small family farm. You may not have access to such a thing, but almost everyone has access to organic meat. Try it. You may find you like the taste even better. You might also like knowing that organic standards demand more humane treatment of the cows, pigs, chickens, turkeys, and egg-laying hens that are slaughtered to make these products.

See if you can work up to a couple of vegetarian meals per week. I've seen families do this in many ways. Some go vegetarian during the week, but then eat meat and/or dairy products on the weekends. Some are vegetarians or vegans until six PM, but have some animal products for dinner. Some quit eating red meat first (beef and pork), then gradually phase out poultry and only eat fish. There are as many ways to do this as there are families, and it all depends on what you want and where you want to go with it.

As you make this transition, you may find that packaged meat substitutes help a lot, and can make the transition much easier. Veggie burgers, veggie sausage, veggie hot dogs, veggie "chicken" nuggets and patties, even veggie barbecued ribs and roasts are all super kid-friendly and can make formerly meat-eating families feel less deprived. These foods are definitely processed. They are not whole foods, so they aren't the ultimate dietary choice, but they are an upgrade. They are better than what they replace, in many ways. Some children I know love veggie burgers and veggie hot dogs, but think "regular" burgers and hot dogs are gross. (I can't help but agree.) These choices might work for you.

But What Do You Eat on Veggie Days?

I've helped so many families make this transition, and many of them are excited about the idea, but when it comes to actually cooking a veggie meal, they panic. What could they possibly make? What would their children *eat*? Many of them are convinced that their children will wither away and die of starvation if they start cooking vegetarian meals.

Mamas, I am here to tell you that this is simply not true. There are many delicious foods children will eat if they get exposed to them regularly—maybe not the first time, maybe not the second time, but maybe the third time. Children also pick up on your hesitation. If you aren't sure about a food, if you don't want to try it, then they probably won't, either. (Or they might be rebellious and demand a larger helping! Hey, maybe we're on to something here. . . .)

They key is to just start making more meals that feature plant foods and meat substitutes, and see what happens. Try black bean burgers, tofu nuggets and tempeh fingers, big colorful salads, warm soups filled with whole grains and tender beans, and the million and one things you can make from nut butter.

Every family is different, so you have to proceed according to what your family will accept, but you also have to move toward what you know is in your family's best interest. If you feel as if your plant foods are a hard sell, just keep it simple and attractive. Who wouldn't be tempted by a bowl of fresh blueberries and strawberries, freshly steamed carrot slices with a little bit of fresh dill and warm butter, sweet potato cubes with a drizzle of maple syrup, or fresh green peas or beans with a sprinkle of salt? Mmm, I'm getting hungry just thinking about it!

Still confused? In the next chapter, I provide simple, easy meal plans that don't include any of the items I've asked you to phase out of your life—they are pure, simple, and free of processed foods, processed sugar, dairy products, and meat, and you can probably make them right now, or with only a few easily obtainable items at your grocery store. Also, see

Organic Nanny Notes

"Nutritional deficiencies! Nutritional deficiencies!" This is the frantic cry often heard by those who feed their children a vegetarian or vegan diet. If you're among them, don't worry, well-meaning mamas. You are not starving your children, even if they tend to be picky eaters! As long as you have plenty of variety, such as beans (including tofu products), pulses such as lentils and peas, whole grains, and nut butters, along with as many different fresh vegetables as possible (especially leafy greens), your child will get plenty of protein and calcium. The only possibility of nutritional deficiencies on a vegan diet containing a variety of organic fruit, vegetables, and whole grains, is vitamin B_{12}, which primarily occurs in animal products. However, this so-called problem is easy to remedy. Just be sure your child has a regular (weekly) source of B_{12} in any of the following:

- A multivitamin with B_{12}
- Cereal fortified with B_{12}
- Tempeh (a yummy fermented soy food with a meaty texture)
- Nutritional yeast (adds cheesy flavor to popcorn and sauces without adding cheese)
- Protein powder fortified with B_{12} (I like the one made by Whole Foods, but there are many other good ones—just read the label to find one without animal residue)

the appendix of this book for a few of my favorite kid-friendly vegetarian recipes, to help get you started.

When you start feeling lighter, cleaner, and more radiant, I suspect you'll be hooked on the veggie lifestyle. But don't take my word for it. Just give it a try, and listen to the wisdom from your own body.

Finally, as with the other letters in L.O.V.E., being veg-centric isn't only about food. Consider animals and vegetables when you buy personal products, shoes, belts, cosmetics, or anything at all. Is the product made from animals, or plants, or petrochemicals? Decide how much it's worth to you. Better to know and ponder than to refuse to see that you are wearing animal skins or using products that were tested on animals.

Many personal products and clothing items are now labeled "vegan," for those who have decided it matters. It's something to think about. (And I just saw the cutest pair of vegan shoes. . . .)

E Is for Environmental

But wait, we have one more letter! The lovely and talented letter E. L.O.V.E. begins locally, and ends globally, because how we care for ourselves and our families and our little communities is a direct reflection of how we care for Mother Earth herself. Every wonderful choice you make can also have one last shading to it: concern for the planet. That's what *E* stands for: Environmental.

As you work through these rules in your own life, you will see how much they begin to intertwine. When you buy locally (*L*), you often end up buying organic (*O*), which is good for the environment (*E*) and eventually may help you feel even more strongly about going veg-centric, vegetarian, or vegan (*V*).

When you go veg-centric, vegetarian, or vegan (*V*), your diet is better for the environment (*E*), and you may recognize that you feel better and cleaner on organic food (*O*), which may be easier to find and less expensive when you buy it locally (*L*).

Do you see how L.O.V.E. is self-perpetuating? Isn't that gorgeous?

Everything you do to build a better life for your children will likely be good for the life of the planet. We are all connected, and it shows. For instance, we don't just believe, we know that industrial animal agriculture is one of the most destructive planetary pollutants. According to the Worldwatch Institute, "The human appetite for animal flesh is a driving force behind virtually every major category of environmental damage now threatening the human future—deforestation, erosion, fresh water scarcity, air and water pollution, climate change, biodiversity loss, social injustice, the destabilization of communities and the spread of disease."

Organic Voices

Don't blow it. Good planets are hard to find.

—*Time* magazine

A recent study also revealed that 51 percent of greenhouse gases produced on the planet come from the livestock industry. That's over half, more than all transportation combined!

This is just one example. Nonlocal food is bad for the environment because it has to be shipped so far to get to its destination, and that means more burning of fossil fuels. Organic food is better for the environment because fewer pesticides and other chemicals enter the environment, and because organic farming is more likely to be concerned with resource preservation. Vegetarian food is better for the animals that won't get eaten, of course, but also because of the aforementioned feedlot statistic. The simple fact is that our food choices not only affect our own health, they affect the health of the very planet we call home.

The good news is that all the other parts of L.O.V.E. contribute to the last part, so you don't really have to do anything in addition if you are already eating locally, organically, and vegan. The letter *E* in L.O.V.E. is pretty much a freebie.

However, there are plenty of other easy little things you can do that aren't directly related to your diet. For example:

- Recycle your junk mail, plastic food containers, and cans. Everyone can participate in filling the recycle bin, or in taking a load to the recycling center and putting recycled items in the correct bins.
- Buy recycled paper products and use fewer paper products such as napkins, paper towels, and toilet paper. Waste not, want not.
- When possible, use real, washable dishes instead of paper and plastic plates, cups, and utensils. The less trash you all make, the better. Get your kids in the habit of rinsing off their own dishes.
- Fix things instead of throwing them away. Break the "Oh well, let's just buy a new one" habit.
- Buy gently used products instead of new products. Consignment stores are so much fun, and often have kids' clothes at bargain prices.
- Bring your own reusable bags to the grocery store. Can your children help you carry them?

Organic Nanny To-Do List

☐ Go local: Visit a farmers' market or roadside produce stand.
☐ Go organic: Try one new organic fruit or vegetable.
☐ Go vegetable-centric, vegetarian, or vegan, at your own pace.
☐ Can you try Meatless Monday?
☐ Go environmental: Do five "green" acts you might not normally do, from recycling or reusing something to walking or biking instead of driving somewhere.
☐ Live with L.O.V.E.: Spend some time this week thinking about other creative ways you could live with L.O.V.E. in your everyday life. Ask your children for their ideas, too.

- Drive less. Walk more and ride a bicycle more. Do it as a family.
- Turn off lights, appliances, televisions, and computers when you aren't using them. Get your kids in the habit, too.
- Pick up trash when you see it. Encourage your children to do so as well. Littering is antiplanet!
- Start a compost pile. Kids can dump the vegetable pairings into it while you make dinner.
- Plant trees in your yard. Let your children help.
- Spend more time outside, with your children, so you gain an increased appreciation for the natural world—it's so easy to forget what's out there, to take it for granted, when you all spend your time inside staring at screens.

In the end, the best, most wonderful thing you can do, for your children, for yourself, for your family, for your community, and for the planet, is to eat with L.O.V.E., live with L.O.V.E., and make L.O.V.E. your mantra. Do you feel the L.O.V.E.? You must, because I can feel it from *here*.

CHAPTER SEVEN

Putting the Pieces Together

I do not like broccoli. I haven't liked it since I was a little kid and my mother made me eat it. I'm president of the United States and I'm not going to eat any more broccoli.

—*George H. W. Bush*

The rule: Don't ask, bribe, or force a child to eat.

—*Dr. Benjamin Spock*, from *Dr. Spock's Baby and Child Care*

*N*ow to the nuts and beans! Families often tell me that they want to eat right but they just don't know how to put the principles into practice. A lot of learning to eat with L.O.V.E. is a matter of trial and error and the willingness to have a sense of adventure, but believe me, Mamas, I know how picky children can be. If your children have been eating junk food and processed food, they also have taste buds accustomed to the simple but overpowering flavors of too much sugar, salt, and fat.

But there are many wonderful ways to get the good stuff into your kids. Gently exposing them to new beautiful foods works some of the time. At other times, and especially with pickier eaters, you may have to employ secret ingredients—clever ways to stash veggies and fruit into food your child already likes. It can be like a game—find all the fun ways to get delicious L.O.V.E. foods into your family's daily diet to help everybody get stronger, healthier, and calmer. Pretty soon, your whole house is going to glow!

An acronym I like to use that encompasses all these strategies is H.E.A.L. Whenever you are serving food, introducing a new food, cooking together, or interacting with your child around food, remember to H.E.A.L.:

H. Hold back on negative words. No bribes, no threats to make your children eat. No child should ever be threatened with a loss of privileges in an attempt to get him to eat. In fact, eating and food should never be associated with any kind of negative experience. Food is food, period. Anything else sets up your children for future eating issues, even an eating disorder.

E. Encourage your children with positive messages. When they eat food you know to be good, show your pleasure. Show your own enjoyment of L.O.V.E. foods. Let the whole eating experience be positive, fun, joyful. Let mealtime be pleasant and relaxed. Be patient with your children. Use cute fun plates and cups. Play music. Have picnics. Food should be fun and healthful!

A. Accept how your children relate to their food. Maybe one child will eat anything. Great! Maybe another tests your patience because she doesn't like to try new things. That is your child. Accept this and work with it instead of telling her she should be someone else. Every child has individual tastes and will interact with food in a unique way.

L. L.O.V.E. foods should make an appearance at every single meal!

Your Picky Eater

I have noticed, over the years, that the way children eat tends to fall into two distinct categories: Adventurers and Testers. Knowing your children's preferences can help a lot as you upgrade your family's diet, because the way your children eat will determine how willing they will be to try new foods—and how creative you will have to be to upgrade their diet.

The Adventurer

Tyler loved to eat, and he would try anything. Mango? Thumbs up. Brussels sprouts? Boiled no, roasted yes. Fruit salad with coconut? Bring it on! He was such a joy to feed because he truly relished food, and never minded if he didn't like something. It wasn't a trauma, it was just something he tried and didn't like. I used to let him try lots of different foods and he would say, "Next course, Nanny!"

Adventurers are born with a strong appetite, and they like to taste everything. They enjoy eating and new foods are unexplored territory to be conquered! With adventurers, you have such a wonderful opportunity to expose them to all the beautiful L.O.V.E. foods you can find. These children may not like them all, but that's fine. They aren't deterred by disliking a taste. Start them early and expose them to everything, so they develop a broad and sophisticated palate.

The only thing to be careful of with Adventurers is to limit fat, salt, and sugar, because a hearty appetite geared toward these simple tastes and high-calorie foods can result in a child who becomes overweight. Just keep an eye on these children's activity level, and keep the L.O.V.E. foods coming! You've got a great opportunity to build a healthy child with ease when you've got an Adventurer.

The Tester

Tyler's little brother, Tim, was a choosy eater, nothing like his brother. When Tyler would try a new food, Tim would screw up his face and seal his lips shut and shake his head adamantly. If he didn't like the look of a food or, heaven forbid, the smell of a food, he wouldn't even *consider* tasting it. He was a real challenge to feed because he had only a few foods he would eat (macaroni and cheese, peanut butter and jelly, and chicken strips), and the rest he would vigorously oppose.

Testers are the choosy eaters. They have a sensitive palate, so new tastes seem more extreme to them. These are the kids who say they don't like a food that they've never even tried. I've seen testers just barely touch their tongue to a forkful of something new, and then recoil in revulsion. They will push food around on their plate for an hour, or find clever ways to get rid of it (many a willing family dog has been an ally to a Tester). I call them Testers because not only do they test foods with their highly specific and choosy standards, but they are likely to test your patience, especially when you are just trying to help them eat better!

Sometimes Testers have food allergies, or they may simply have more reactive or sensitive taste buds. Some of these children can be very thin because they don't eat very much. Some can become overweight because they only like a few high-fat, high-sugar foods, and they overeat those foods. For these little ones, you have to be more creative by finding more appealing ways to serve healthy food. For example, vegetable and fruit purees can be added to many comfort foods Testers already like. They may not even notice the difference.

Understanding what kind of eater your child is will help prepare you for the best ways to feed her. Remember the *A* in H.E.A.L.: accept. Accept what kind of eater your child is, and work with it, rather than trying to change her into something she's not.

Now that you have a strategy and a clear idea about what you are up against as you begin your quest to phase out processed foods, sugar, white flour, dairy, and meat, and phase in more plant foods, let's start with our babies when they are, well . . . still babies.

Feeding Babies with L.O.V.E.

If your child is still a baby and just beginning to eat solid food, you are in the best possible position to develop your baby's healthy eating habits. This is the time to introduce the very best foods, and leave the bad stuff out of the picture entirely. You may even be able to encourage a natural Tester to be more adventurous by exposing her to many different tastes in the second half of her first year, and on through the toddler years. Even

No-No Foods

Babies should not be introduced to solid food before four months of age, and many pediatricians say that they can benefit from six full months of breastfeeding before the introduction of solid foods. Once babies do start eating, recommendations differ on the foods that they should not eat before a certain age. Talk to your pediatrician to get individual recommendations. Generally, these are the foods that some pediatricians say babies should not eat before the age of six months, or up to one or even two years:

- *Honey, because of the risk of botulism.* Virtually everyone agrees no baby should be exposed to honey before one year of age.
- *Peanuts, nuts, and their butters.* Recommendations vary from six months to two years. You might as well wait. Peanut and nut allergies can be quite serious.
- *Broccoli, beans, and other gas-producing foods.* Some doctors say to wait on these foods just because a gassy baby is a very loud and uncomfortable baby. Some babies don't have a problem with these foods, however. Many older babies approaching their first birthday enjoy them, especially beans.
- *Strawberries.* Some children are highly allergic to strawberries, so avoid these until your child is at least one year old. Blueberry puree is fine for younger children.
- *Egg whites.* Recommendations vary from six to twelve months.
- *Cow's milk.* Most pediatricians agree that no child should drink cow's milk until after the age of one year. (I suggest it be avoided forever.) Goat's milk can be easier for many children to digest, but if you want to try this, wait until after they are one year old.
- *Wheat.* Recommendations vary from six months to one year. Start babies on gentler grains, like brown rice, whole oats, and barley.
- *Shellfish.* I don't think children ever need to eat shellfish, but if your child wants to try it, wait until your baby is at least one year old.
- *Soy.* Many children drink soy formula as infants, but it doesn't agree with some, so if a doctor recommends avoiding soy, please do so.

babies express preferences, but those preferences can change from day to day, moment to moment. A ten-month-old who doesn't like pureed spinach or carrots one day may gobble it up the next, so keep trying different fruit and vegetables in particular.

At about five or six months, begin introducing your baby to the simple, pure tastes of organic vegetables and fruit. You can make these yourself by gently steaming organic produce and then pureeing it in your own blender with a little bit of purified water. So simple and easy! This is the ultimate baby food. You can make big batches of homemade baby food and freeze it in ice cube trays. Or, especially when you are pressed for time, you can purchase organic baby food.

Begin with vegetables, so your baby doesn't learn immediately to prefer sweet tastes over savory. After your baby has tried a few different vegetables—for example, pureed squash, carrots, peas, green beans, and avocado—try introducing a few simple fruit—pureed peaches, plums, apples, and blueberries. After your baby is enjoying vegetables and fruit, try introducing organic whole-grain cereals, such as brown rice cereal, and silken tofu.

Introduce tastes, one per day or one per week, and see what your baby loves. Try a puree of green beans one day, apricots the next, then butternut squash, then banana, then a porridge of brown rice—or just puree one of the fruit, vegetables, or grains you are eating. Keep the processed food, sugar, and white flour products out of the picture entirely, and don't even bother with the meat and dairy. The rainbow of plant foods out there is all your baby needs. As your baby gets older, you can start mixing foods, or pureeing more complex dishes that you are eating. After nine or ten months, try vegetarian refried beans, pureed lasagne, guacamole, or a pureed homemade stir-fry.

Organic Voices

Pick battles big enough to matter and small enough to win.

—*Jonathan Kozol*

Your baby's food should be made from foods you choose with the same high standards you use to choose foods for yourself. The fresher, the better. Organic produce from the farmers' market is an excellent choice. Or grow a baby food garden with carrots, peas, beans, summer and winter squashes, and corn.

Feeding Toddlers

Once your child is a toddler, the options become so much more exciting. You don't have to puree everything anymore (although you might still choose to do that, as many older kids enjoy the comforting nature of a puree). Toddlers are champion snackers, so make sure you've got plenty of soft, yummy, finger food around. They can become randomly choosy or open to different foods, so the best thing to do is keep trying different foods, including the ones they've previously rejected, and always keep the eating experience fun and positive. No guilt, no pressure, just yummy food with Mommy!

Some L.O.V.E. foods to try (get organic whenever possible):

- Avocado cubes
- Pear slices
- Silken tofu and baked tofu cubes
- Banana wheels
- Diced apple
- Soft-cooked carrot slices
- Cooked green peas
- Canned white or black beans (drain canned beans and rinse first to remove salty liquid)
- Little pieces of fresh tomato
- Cooked sweet potato cubes
- Dry whole-grain cereals (without added sugar—read the label!)

You can also let your toddler practice using a spoon by offering:

- Applesauce
- Oatmeal

About Breastfeeding

You can probably already guess what I think about breastfeeding: it's the best! Breastfeeding offers so many health benefits to babies, and such a close and intimate bonding experience between mother and child, that I highly recommend every mother at least give it a try, and try to breastfeed for at least a few months. I know it doesn't work for every family, and that's okay. Better to be a good mama who isn't saddled with guilt just because you didn't breastfeed. If it does work for you, however, then super!

Even after you introduce your baby to solid foods, you can breastfeed for several years as a supplement to your child's increasingly diverse diet. You and your baby will know when it's time to wean. Don't let anyone else tell you that they know better than you do.

- Butternut squash soup
- Mashed potatoes
- Cream of rice or wheat cereal

These are just a tiny toddler handful of ideas. Just keep experimenting and building on the foods your toddler loves. Be he an Adventurer or Tester, as long as it's fresh, natural, and organic, your child just might love it. If you don't offer it, you'll never know. And neither will he.

Preschool and Beyond: Menus for Childhood

Once your child is old enough to eat just about anything, the real fun begins. This is the age of family dinners, visits to the farmers' market, picnics in the park, gardening, and creative sack lunches. This is the childhood they will remember, so everything you do surrounding food will make an impression on your child for many years to come.

Now, don't be nervous. You've got the Organic Nanny to help you. I promised you some simple easy kid-friendly menus in the last chapter—menus that don't include processed foods, sugar, white flour, dairy products, eggs, or meat, and which are brimming with vitamins, minerals, fiber, protein, complex carbohydrates and healthy fats.

Try following this menu for a week, or follow a close approximation of it, just to see how your kids respond. These are just ideas. Customize for what your kids like, or experiment with new foods to get them interested. You can substitute any meal in a column for any other, or just make something similar.

As you go through the week feeding your children this healthful menu of real whole plant foods, watch for changes in behavior, weight, energy, and health. I predict great things for your children, Mamas. After the first week, you will be ready to go it on your own, exploring the wonderful world of plant foods in a veg-centric reverie. Or, just do this week again, with a few more variations.

Notes on the menu:
- *Butter* means a trans-fat-free, dairy-free buttery spread, such as Earth Balance.
- *Milk* means any plant milk, such as soy, rice, almond, or coconut milk.
- *Cheese* means vegan cheese, such as Follow Your Heart or Daiya brands.
- When I mention a product such as peanut butter or applesauce, I mean the natural types, without added sugar.
- Don't worry about portion size. With foods like these, your child should be able to eat until she is satisfied without overeating. A child's hunger level varies from day to day. Respect her natural rhythms.
- Meals with an asterisk (*) have corresponding recipes at the end of this book.

The Lost Art of Cooking

This menu isn't the end of the story. Life extends far beyond a seven-day menu, so let's talk about some of the other ways to feed your kids with L.O.V.E., as well as with love. First and foremost, I want to talk about cooking.

	BREAKFAST	SNACK	LUNCH	SNACK	DINNER
MONDAY	Mango cubes and banana slices Rice milk	Simple Guacamole* with corn chips	Veggie burgers on whole-grain buns Homemade French Fries*	Orange Slices with Cinnamon Cream*	Tofu Fingers* Corn on the cob Green Salad*
TUESDAY	Orange-Strawberry Smoothie* Whole-grain toast with peanut butter	Hummus* with whole-grain pita triangles	Whole wheat pasta with butter and sea salt, green beans	Nicki's Almond Nut Butter Boats*	Organic Nanny Tacos* Cuban Salsa*
WEDNESDAY	Fried Tofu Breakfast Sandwich* Fresh blueberries	Leftover Cuban Salsa with corn chips	Whole wheat toast with almond or peanut butter and banana slices drizzled with maple syrup	Carrot sticks or cherry tomatoes with cubes of vegan cheese (e.g., Follow Your Heart mozzarella)	Make-Your-Own-Pizzas* (or try Amy's brand vegan and gluten-free options, or Tofurkey brand. Green salad
THURSDAY	Oatmeal with real maple syrup and rice milk Freshly squeezed orange juice	Edamame with salt	Peanut Butter Roll-Ups* Pear slices	Frozen juice pops	Pasta with Red Sauce* Whole-Grain Garlic Bread* Green salad

	Breakfast	Snack	Lunch	Snack	Dinner
FRIDAY	Blueberry Pancakes with Strawberry Sauce*	Celery sticks with peanut butter and raisins	Soup—choose your child's favorite kind (bean, pea, noodle, tomato) or make your own favorite (Amy's brand makes many good ones.) Melon slices	Larabar	Tata's Cuban Rice with Secret Sofrito* Cuban Mashed Sweet Potatoes* Green Salad* L.O.V.E. Cupcakes*
SATURDAY	Purple Power Smoothie* Optional: Veggie sausage patty (Lightlife Gimme Lean sausage is vegan.)	Coconut or pecan date rolls (Tierra Farm makes good ones that are organic.)	Grilled PB&J* Baby carrots with Hummus* for dipping	Whole-grain crackers with Hummus* Mango slices	Tempeh fingers (Slice tempeh, brush with soy sauce, and fry.) Organic Nanny Mashed Potatoes* Steamed green beans with butter
SUNDAY	L.O.V.E. Muffins* Chocolate rice milk	Organic grapes	Bean Burritos* Guacamole	Magic Mix*	Noodles with butter Green salad

Meals with an asterisk (*) have corresponding recipes in Appendix One, beginning on page 225.

Over the last twenty years, it has been my good fortune to work with children from an economically diversified and multicultural cross-section of the population; and being exposed to so many different types of families, I've noticed something interesting: The wealthiest people and the poorest share something in common—they eat a lot of processed foods, and in general have no clue what to do with whole foods such as whole grains, beans, and fresh produce. If it doesn't come in a box with a picture on it and specific microwave instructions, they are lost.

It amazes me how few people cook anymore.

I suppose it's no surprise—people who are the poorest and the wealthiest tend to have the most stress and the least time and energy for cooking as a hobby. Many people I've encountered say they hate to cook, or they don't have time, or they just don't know how. Oh, the exquisite kitchens I've seen that never get used!

I think what most people who say they don't like to cook don't realize is that cooking doesn't have to be complicated or messy or time consuming. Kids prefer simple foods anyway, and often, the simplest foods are the most nutritious. Learning some very basic cooking skills and sharing them with your children is not just a fun pursuit, but a great way to relieve stress and get healthier, less-processed food into your child's diet and life. Cooking provides time for bonding with your child and it teaches many helpful skills as you read directions together, measure out ingredients, and watch food transform from its raw state to something you made together. Choosy eaters tend to be much more interested in trying a food they helped prepare, or a snack they made themselves.

You might even instill a lifelong interest in cooking healthy food.

Recently, I taught a cooking class for children at a school, where I met a bunch of great parents who were educated and wanted to make healthy choices for their families, but they were full of questions because they really weren't sure exactly what was healthy and what wasn't. I explained to them that if it's fresh and whole, it's healthy. Then, all they have to do is learn how to prepare it. When it comes to kids, simpler is usually better, and cooking whole foods simply is really pretty easy and quick.

Slow Down and Relish the Table

I've noticed something interesting about families with busy, stressed-out parents. Many of these mamas and papas wolf down their food quickly, so they can move on to the next order of business. I've noticed that in these situations, the children often sit at the table refusing to eat. Of course, this frustrates already stressed-out parents even more. You are in a hurry, and now your child is balking at eating a slice of pizza, for goodness' sake?

I believe children do this, consciously or unconsciously, as a way to protest the stressful, hurried vibe they are getting from their parents. Mealtime should be a relaxed, happy time. It's not a time for wolfing down food and rushing off, and it's not a time for arguing or bringing up sensitive issues, like, "Here's your salad, honey, and what's up with that D you got in biology?"

The happiest, best memories of family meals are of happy times when everybody laughs and eats peacefully and even lingers for a few minutes for prolonged conversation before clearing away the dishes.

A papa recently told me, "I don't remember any of the fast food meals I ate as a child, but I remember the meals at the table with my family. Those are great memories."

You are making those memories right now, so make them a priority. I know that sometimes, you will have a tight schedule and you will have to hurry off, but let that be the exception, not the rule. Family dinner matters. Prove it to your children. If they are used to eating and running or eating in front of the television, you may need to go gradually. Eat at the table one night per week at first, then two, then three. Even a few family meals every week make a difference in a child's grades, self-esteem, and behavior. I can guarantee you won't regret it.

A good place to start is with the recipes at the end of this book. But there is so much more to learn! I've found some absolutely excellent vegan cookbooks out there that will tell you all the basics you need to know. Some are geared toward kids and some aren't, but they all contain simple, healthful, natural recipes centered around plant foods. You can also find all over the Internet tons of great information on cooking plant foods. The resources appendix at the end of this book will guide you toward some of the books and Web sites I use and love.

The best thing you can do is just get back in the kitchen. Don't be afraid! You are modeling healthy food-related behavior around your children when you go in there and start working with food. Better yet, they can help you. Children who learn to help cook from an early age tend to be more adventurous and curious eaters, and children have a natural affinity for food. Make the most of it now, while they are still interested.

Stealth Health

Now let's talk about another issue—let's go back to those Testers. You can kid-friendly-up your menus all you want, but sometimes, it's not going to work. They *know* they haven't had those strange foods before, and they have no intention of budging. Does this sound familiar? (If it doesn't, you are one lucky mama!)

Let's be frank, Mamas. Sometimes, everybody loves the dinner you made, but sometimes, especially in a house full of Testers, your child just isn't going to eat those leafy greens, or zucchini slices, or whatever it is you labored over with so much love. Sometimes they may even resist the things you were sure they would love—who doesn't like blueberries, bananas, baby carrots? Maybe your child doesn't. There isn't any point in arguing about it. Your child is who she is, and that deserves respect.

I would never condone lying to a child, but you also have the very important job of feeding your children a healthy diet. The answer I've found that works best is to include Secret Agent Ingredients in the foods you cook for your family.

My favorite way to do this is to make purees. Keep your blender handy, because purees can slide into so many different foods unnoticed—it's stealth health!

Fruit purees have a sweet pleasant taste, so they are easy to incorporate into baked goods such as muffins, cookies, and cupcakes. Try purees of fresh blueberries, raspberries, and strawberries (strain out the seeds if you think that will bother your child). Other good fruit purees include apple, pear, banana, and orange. Fruit purees can also substitute for some of the fat in baked goods.

Vegetable purees can hide in your child's favorite food like a ninja, upping the nutritional content without engendering a single "Yucky!" I have some core vegetable purees I like to add to many basic recipes. Trust me, nannies have been doing this for many years! Make this a habit—a fruit or vegetable in every cooked dish!

The best way to engage in stealth health is to make a batch of fruit puree and a batch of vegetable puree every weekend. Keep them in the refrigerator in a jar, and pour or scoop out the puree into your child's food all week long. Base your purees on whatever fruit and vegetables are fresh and in season—and always use organic if you can.

Here are some ways I like to use purees. Try these, or invent your own clever nutrient infusions:

- Add butternut squash, pumpkin, or carrot puree (or a combination) to yellow and red foods, such as macaroni and cheese, pizza sauce, pasta sauce, or even into applesauce or vanilla yogurt.
- Add cauliflower puree to mashed potatoes or noodle soup.
- Add a leaf of fresh kale to a fruit smoothie. (Start with a small amount and gradually increase the greens-to-fruit ratio.) Smoothies should be very sweet, very cold, and an appealing color when you first introduce them to a child. Think: ice cream–like. (See the next section for more about smoothies.)
- Puree any soft steamed vegetable, such as broccoli, green beans, or peas. Add them in small amounts to anything, from chili to cupcakes!
- I also like to add Cuban flavor to my dishes. Kids are naturally attracted to the flavors of Cuban cuisine because they are mild and sweet. I like to add purees of mango, pineapple, avocado, papaya, and sweet potato. Delicious! (See the recipes at the end of this book for some of my Cuban favorites.)

When you add fruit and vegetable purees to your children's pasta or banana bread or even their chocolate brownies, you are adding fiber and nutrients, antioxidants and vitamins and minerals, to replace all those chemically altered ingredients in processed foods. This is an excellent way to start upgrading the foods you are eating as you are phasing out less healthy choices. As a bonus, these ingredients will help your children digest their food better (because of the fiber) and will not contribute to overeating (because of the lack of appetite-charging processed ingredients).

Magical Juices and Super-Power Smoothies

Another way to get the good stuff into kids is to begin juicing. It's also one of the best and most effective ways to incorporate secret ingredients into your child's diet. Most kids will drink delicious freshly squeezed juice or a freshly blended smoothie. Most children automatically like the sweet taste of fruit, especially familiar produce such as apples or oranges. It's only a small step to get them to try homemade juice, especially when you start with sweet ones, and work in other ingredients as your child gets curious.

As for smoothies, I believe a daily smoothie is a potentially dramatic health-enhancing habit that every child can grow to love. Smoothies and juices are an easy sell because they are familiar—they look like sugary drinks and ice cream, but they are so much better. Even if your children balk at first, persistence is the ticket.

With smoothies and juices in your arsenal, you've got some powerful tools for building healthy kids. I once cared for a little girl, Emily, who was five years old. She wasn't at all sure she wanted to drink her first smoothie, so she told me, "I bet the dog won't even eat it!" I said, "Well, let's pour her a bowl of smoothie and see if she likes it."

Sure enough, that dog lapped up every drop. Emily decided if the dog liked it, it must be good. She's been a happy smoothie consumer ever since. (And that was a big "Whew!" for me, because I really wasn't sure whether the dog would like it! Thanks, puppy, for your help!)

To make fresh juice, I highly recommend purchasing a quality juicer that is easy to clean and will stand up to daily use. The Total Blender by

Smoothie "Medicine"

Another great use for smoothies is to provide extra nutrition when a child is sick. Sick children often don't want to eat, but they will drink something. Smoothies can also help with constipation because the fiber in the fruit softens the bowels. Add flaxseed oil to a bedtime smoothie for a gentle overnight laxative effect—no cramps, no drugs. Add protein powder and/or a spoonful of almond butter to a morning smoothie for a dose of protein to keep your child nourished and energetic throughout the day. For children who need to put on a little bit of weight, nut butters make an excellent addition to smoothies.

Blendtec is my favorite. Some prefer the Vitamix. Both make juice and smoothies. Or, if you already have a blender and a juicer, those are fine, too. Juice and smoothies make good snacks as well as breakfasts.

You can find my juice and smoothie recipes at the back of this book.

Once your child has gotten into the juice-and-smoothie habit, get creative together. Very gradually increase the proportion of leafy greens to fruit (ideally you will work up to half greens, half fruit), but keep it yummy. If your child doesn't like it, back off on the green stuff a bit. Remember, never force your child to eat! Better to throw away a bad batch of juice or smoothie than create tension and negative feelings about food.

Special additions that can make the smoothie even sweeter:

- 1 teaspoon unsweetened cocoa powder or raw cacao nibs
- Pinch of cinnamon
- Drop of vanilla extract or other flavored extract.
- 1 teaspoon ground flaxseed or flaxseed oil
- 1 teaspoon raw wheat germ
- 1 tablespoon peanut or nut butter (e.g., almond, cashew)
- Any other fresh or frozen fruit you happen to have on hand

Sensational Snacks

Kids love snacks, so snack time is another great way to upgrade your child's diet. Let's say it's family movie night, or your kids are having a sleepover at your house. You've got a house full of preteen girls or grade school boys running wildly about, and you are just getting ready to break out the chips and corn puffs and packaged cookies to appease the natives, aren't you? Oh no, don't tell me you even bought a bag of candy!

Of course, it's what the kids want, especially if that's the custom. However, there are other options, options that might even calm down that crew a bit. Instead of junk food snacks, you can stock your cupboards with easy-to-grab goodies that won't harm your child's health. How about:

- Whole-grain crackers and pretzels
- Veggie chips (sweet potato chips, yum!)
- Apple slices with peanut butter for dipping
- A big bowl of fresh grapes or blueberries (kids devour these!)
- Organic fruit snacks
- Whole-grain, naturally sweetened cookies or cupcakes (even better if you made them yourself!)
- Trail mix—make your own with fresh organic dried fruit (raisins, naturally sweetened cranberries, snipped apricots) and peanuts, almonds, walnuts, or other favorite nuts. A few vegan chocolate chips make it even more appealing.
- Dried apricots, dried banana chips, dried apple rings—dried fruit is like candy, but so much better!
- Pickles on sticks
- Celery with almond butter
- Edamame
- Pitted olives
- Sweet red pepper strips, baby carrots, and whole-grain pita triangles with hummus dip

The Yeast You Need to Know

Nutritional yeast is a vegan staple because it adds a cheesy flavor to foods, without the actual cheese. Don't confuse nutritional yeast with the kind of yeast you would use to bake bread. They are completely different. Nutritional yeast is an edible product similar to brewer's yeast, available in health food stores. It is a flaky sort of powder and many vegan recipes use it as an ingredient for things like macaroni and "cheese" or scrambled tofu. It also makes an excellent topping for popcorn. Why not give it a try? It's really good.

- Baked tortilla chips and organic purchased or homemade salsa or pico de gallo
- Fresh popcorn sprinkled with a little sea salt and garlic or onion powder, and/or a sprinkle of nutritional yeast, instead of butter

Trust me—if it's a snack and it's in a bowl, the kids are going to eat it.

And what about the ultimate snack: plain old fruit and vegetables. All you have to do is spend a few minutes cutting it up. Make this a weekly habit: Cut up vegetables for a tray with dip, and cut up fruit or prepare it so it's ready to eat from a fruit bowl. After school, put out the trays and bowls and let them go at it. Try hummus dip or white bean dip, salsa, or guacamole. Dipping foods is fun, and if it's there and the kids are hungry, they won't go foraging for the junk food. You might be shocked at how eagerly they attack the fresh stuff. Their bodies hone in on it and know they need it.

I used to nanny for a family with three little girls. The next-door neighbor was a little boy named Jeremy, and I don't think he was given very much fresh food because, every day after school, he would come over and linger in the kitchen, watching me, until I put out the fruit and vegetables. You should have seen this little guy eat, as if he'd never had a piece of fruit in his life! The girls would watch with amusement as they picked at grapes

> ## *Organic Nanny Notes*
>
> Mamas, do you know why your child loves all those neon-colored snacks? It's because they contain seasoning blends with a mix of artificial colors and flavors, often including monosodium glutamate (MSG). These flavors have been created by food scientists to extend shelf life and to get your kids to eat more by enhancing the addictive quality. This is why you "can't eat just one." You get that taste in your mouth and you have to keep going!
>
> Would your child binge on celery or orange slices? Probably not. But chips? Oh yes, I've seen it a hundred times. MSG interferes with the production of leptin, a hormone that helps regulate the appetite. Feed it to your kids, and they don't have a chance. Instead of serving junk food filled with fake ingredients, look for similar items, such as natural tortilla chips flavored with natural ingredients. I love Garden of Eatin' baked blue corn chips. Served with a yummy homemade dip, salsa, or guacamole, it should fill in the gap, and help restore your child's natural appetite.

or celery sticks and he would polish off the rest of the tray. The youngest girl, a sweetie named Laura, once said to me, "Nanny, I think Jeremy needs to come to our house so he can be healthy!" I think she was right.

Sure, eating and snacking like this takes a tiny bit more effort. The best things always do. Your kids may whine at first when they can't find the toaster pastries and the ranch-flavored chips and bags of candy in the first few seconds they think they desire those foods, but once they begin to feel better and you start to see a change in their looks, behavior, and energy levels, there will be no turning back. When your child looks at you with rosy cheeks and asks for more apple slices, you'll have all the reward you ever needed.

L.O.V.E. Food All Day Long

Feeding kids L.O.V.E. foods takes a little practice, it's true, but look how well you are doing already! With gradual changes and lots of positive attitude from the grown-ups in the house, your kids will come around. Be patient and remember to slow down and make positive changes where you can—a few at first, then a few more. Do your best! Here are just a few more inspiring ideas for regular mealtimes:

- Serve a big, fresh salad with colorful raw vegetables at every meal. If ranch or another dressing helps them eat it, find or make a natural organic version, then pour it on!
- In winter, make hearty, chunky soups. Keep the familiar foods coming, but upgrade them.
- Make noodles of all types—spaghetti, elbow macaroni, penne, rice noodles—whole grains are great, or mix regular with some whole-grain pasta at first, until everyone gets used to the heartier taste. Top with your favorite pasta sauce, or just a little bit of trans-fat-free margarine. Remember to add veggie purees to your pasta sauces.
- Whole-grain tortillas made into quesadillas, burritos, or tostadas make delicious, customizable meals. Fill or top with whatever your child likes. Try vegetarian refried beans, a little bit of nondairy cheese, and a few favorite vegetables such as tomatoes, corn, or shredded carrots. Or, fill taco shells with anything, from Mexican-flavored veggie "crumbles" (resembles ground beef) to soft white or black beans, shredded lettuce, chopped tomatoes, vegan cheese shreds, and avocado. Also try olives, shredded cabbage, or nontraditional taco fillings your kids might like, such as green peas, corn, cubed potatoes, or chopped broccoli. Tacos are like a blank slate just waiting for you to be creative.
- Pizza is another great palette ready for your ingenuity. Make your own with a whole-grain crust, organic tomato sauce (with added veggie purees), and one or two favorite veggies. You can even buy vegan "pepperoni"!
- Upgrade grilled "cheese" made with vegan cheese and olive oil or trans-fat-free spread. Add any veggies your child likes. Mushrooms? Tomato slices? Avocado? Experiment. If your child likes tomato soup, add a bowl for dipping.

Your Child: The Remix

When a child switches from an animal-based and processed food diet to a whole-food, plant-based diet, these are the changes I have seen firsthand:

- A healthy glow
- Quicker healing of cuts and bruises
- Better sleep
- Sweeter breath
- Less tooth decay, fewer cavities
- Clear skin
- More energy
- Fewer colds

- Many kids enjoy tofu fingers or nuggets rolled in whole-grain rice cereal and baked until crispy. They're like fast-food chicken strips, but so much better! Serve with a creamy dipping sauce made from half vegan mayonnaise and half naturally sweetened ketchup (high in healthy lycopene), barbecue sauce, or mustard. (See the recipe for Tofu Fingers at the end of this book.)
- A fun food to eat is grilled vegetables and tofu cubes on a stick with peanut sauce (mix peanut butter with water and a bit of soy sauce and maple syrup).
- Baked beans make an excellent, protein- and fiber-rich filling on baked potatoes or mashed sweet potatoes.
- A quick weeknight staple: veggie burgers with lettuce and tomato, and baked sweet potato fries with maple syrup for dipping
- Try breakfast for dinner: whole-grain waffles with fresh fruit puree and veggie sausages.
- Applesauce or maple-sweetened pumpkin puree layered with soy or coconut yogurt and berries makes a pretty and delicious parfait for dessert.

The possibilities are endless when you cook and serve food with L.O.V.E. For more ideas on what to cook for your kids with complete recipes, turn to the end of this book.

Final Lesson:
For the Sake of Your Child, Be in Charge!

Mamas, let me take your hands (metaphorically, of course), and tell you something, nanny to mama. You are doing your best. I know that. Parenting is hard, and changing habits is perhaps even harder. When you are feeling stressed, slow down and breathe (and check out Chapter 9).

Also, I want you to remember how powerful and influential you are in your child's life. You are glowing with loving, compassionate authority. Your children may try to boss you around sometimes, as they test their boundaries, and sometimes, you might feel as if you can't possibly say no to them, but I would like to remind you of something very important: You are in charge, and deep down, you know that. You are strong and capable and you know, better than any small child, what is best.

Sometimes, this is easy for mamas to forget. When it comes to meals (and bedtime), I can't tell you how often I see the kids running the show. You are tired, you've had a long day, and you don't feel like fighting with your kids about what to eat. I completely understand how this feels.

However, if you have decided that you are going to feed your children better, you have to stick to it, no matter what. You don't have to make the absolute best choice every single time for every single meal, but don't give up, Mamas. There is too much at stake. This is your organic promise to your babies. Model good eating behavior, and insist on it for everyone who lives in your home.

When the going gets stressful, it may help to remind yourself that you are strong and powerful and you know more than you might always realize. You have a powerful intuition and a halo of loving energy. Your job isn't to give your children only things they like. It's to raise them well and help them learn how to be healthy, so eventually they can venture out into the world on their own and stay healthy. They need your respect

Organic Nanny To-Do List

☐ Try some or all of the meals in the Organic Nanny Meal Plan.
☐ Venture back into the kitchen and try making something from scratch that you usually buy in a more processed form.
☐ Make a smoothie and share it with everyone. Get their opinions on how to tweak the recipe.
☐ Make a fruit or veggie puree and sneak it into a food your kids like, such as macaroni and cheese or spaghetti. Does anybody notice?
☐ Serve healthy snacks all week.
☐ Be in charge!

and your guidance, your love and your leadership. Your job is to teach them how to live . . . and eat . . . without you someday.

You know that, but I know that sometimes it helps to be reminded.

Someday, they will look back fondly on these times and say things like, "Oh, my mom was so crazy with her health food! Pass the salad, please."

Be the parent they will thank, the one whose good advice they will someday appreciate when they are wise adults, even if they don't appreciate it now. Imagine your child as an adult someday, thinking to herself, "Hmm, you know, my mom was right." Sweet victory!

CHAPTER EIGHT

Detoxing Your Home

When you're green inside, you're clean inside.

—Dr. Bernard Jensen

*W*hen Anne and Tom got the news that they were going to have a baby, nobody had to tell them to go organic. They immediately decided to switch everything in their lives to organic—even the nanny!

When they first called me, Anne was insistent, as if she had to convince me that organic was better: "This isn't just the polar ice caps we're talking about. This is our baby. Our child's life is at stake. Everything is full of chemicals! You have to help us get ready!"

Of course I said I would, but when I came to their home to consult with them about child-proofing and detoxifying the house before the baby arrived, I saw that I had a lot to do. Anne and Tom thought they were doing everything right, but they had no idea how much they were missing in their quest to make their home organic.

As you polish up your family's diet, as the toxins start to come out and you all start to feel cleaner and purer and more energetic and just better, you will begin to see how powerful true health can be. But what you eat, although a huge part of health, isn't the only part. To live a truly organic lifestyle, you must also consider where you live, what you

---

Organic Nanny Alert!

When you are pregnant, everything you eat, drink, breathe, and put on your skin could potentially reach your baby as she grows inside of you. Keep your insides and outsides as pure as possible during this sensitive and lovely time.

---

breathe, what you bathe in, what you put on your skin, and even how the products you use affect your home in a larger sense—the planet you live on.

Unfortunately, the world is full of toxins. We use them to clean ourselves, our children, and our homes. We spray them on our lawns and fill our sinks and tubs with them. And don't even get me started about what's floating around in the air and the groundwater—and where are our little ones? Crawling around on those chemically cleaned carpets and chemically slicked floors, bathing in those chemical-filled tubs and playing on those chemically sprayed lawns. Breathing the air, drinking the water, living on the planet that frankly, the human race isn't treating very well. Ave Maria Purisima!

If the toxins in our environment are harmful to adults—and we know from countless studies that they are—then just imagine how harmful they are to our sensitive children, our infants, our unborn babies, even our little pets, and all the other animals that live and breathe and swim and fly in the natural world.

According to Healthy Child, Healthy World, a nonprofit organization dedicated to educating parents about chemical exposure and the risk to children (check out their Web site, www.healthychild.org), you should know these startling facts:

- Exposure to pesticides, hazardous air pollutants, and formaldehyde increases the risk of childhood cancers.
- Poor indoor air quality is a major contributor to the rapid rise in childhood asthma, particularly in preschool-aged children.

- Many chemicals in our environment, including lead, mercury, PCBs, alcohol, and solvents, are known to affect brain development and could be triggers or causes for autism and ADHD, which are rapidly increasing in children.
- According to the Environmental Protection Agency, up to 600,000 children born each year in the United States suffer a mild to moderate loss of IQ points due to methyl mercury exposure during fetal development, mostly from consumption of fish.
- The average newborn's umbilical cord blood contains an average of two hundred chemicals and pollutants from the environment.
- When a pregnant woman is exposed to secondhand tobacco smoke, chemicals in the smoke, including nicotine, can cross the placenta and may lead to birth defects or low birth rate.
- According to one study, babies born to mothers who frequently used chemical cleaners were twice as likely to develop breathing problems.
- Ten percent of calls to the U.S. Poison Control Center involve toxic exposure to household cleaners, and two-thirds of those calls involve children.
- The average American household contains sixty-three different hazardous chemical products, equal to about ten gallons of hazardous waste.

Yikes, Mamas! That's enough to make any of us jump right in with Anne and Tom and start detoxing our homes. I don't want to scare you but I do want to spur you on to action. Too many children have developed serious health problems, in childhood or later in their lives, because of chemical exposure. We must do our part to make sure your children remain safe from this kind of harm!

Organic Voices

For the first time in the history of the world, every human being is now subjected to contact with dangerous chemicals, from the moment of conception until death.

—*Rachel Carson*,
from the book *Silent Spring*

So let's take action! I want to help you get as many of these toxins out of your child's environment as possible. And while we're at it, we might as well do our part to help clean up the planet, too. Because after all, this is the Earth your babies will someday inherit.

Detoxing your home is the beginning. When you take a few simple steps to reduce your chemical use and exposure, you can drastically improve your child's current and future health. I can think of no better reason than that to start right now. It won't even be hard, I promise!

Indoor Air Pollution

Most families probably don't realize just how toxic their homes are, especially when they are remodeling. Many of these toxins hang in the air we breathe, or lie waiting on the surfaces where we sit and lounge, especially where we sleep.

For example, Papa Tom had painted the nursery, to his wife's specifications, in a beautiful blue. However, they didn't realize that most conventional paint off-gasses nasty fumes. (Off-gassing, sometimes called outgassing, is the release of gases into the air due to volatile organic compounds [VOCs] in materials and liquids such as household cleaners, paint, new carpet, and building materials—this creates indoor air pollution.) Meanwhile, Anne had bought all kinds of pretty baby things, such as cute light blue baby sheets with little yellow ducks—a product that was treated in flame-retardants and other chemicals.

The cozy baby mattress was bleached and chemically treated. The new carpet, while beautiful and cozy, was also releasing chemicals into the air. After a cup of calming tea and a tour of their home, I sat down with Mama Anne and Papa Tom and broke the bad news: The new baby's room was off-gassing like crazy! This was no place for a newborn.

Then I gave them a list of changes, which I hope you will also consider for your own child's room—and for your room as well:

- Purchase a new organic mattress made of all-natural materials. Ditch the polyester pillows and bedding, too. Go for natural materials. Check out a company called www.nontoxic.com if you can't find these products in your town. Also check out www.serenitypillows .com.

- Get rid of the spray-painted crib or bed frame and purchase an organic, sustainable, untreated hardwood crib and other furniture, such as baby dressers, changing tables, and rockers.
- Use nontoxic, VOC-free paint every time you ever paint anything in your home! That applies to walls and furniture, too.
- Limit houseplants. While they can clean the air, they must be meticulously maintained to prevent mold growth. New parents in particular probably don't have time to be thinking about the houseplants.
- When replacing carpets and curtains, buy those made of untreated natural materials, such as organic cotton, wool, or hemp. Better yet, lose the carpets completely because all carpets outgas to some extent, and even natural carpets are typically adhered with an off-gassing carpet adhesive. More benign flooring options include natural hardwood, bamboo, ceramic tile, or natural cork flooring. Cover natural hardwood floors with simple rugs made from natural materials, and hang bamboo shades over the windows.
- In bedrooms and the nursery, install an air purifier that uses a genuine HEPA air cleaner. This will dramatically improve the air quality in rooms where we all spend so much time breathing deeply.
- Install a high-efficiency, disposable furnace filter and change it every two to three months. Upgrading your furnace filter will improve the air quality throughout the entire house. Choose one with an 11 or 12 MERV (Minimum Efficiency Reporting Value) rating.
- Open windows whenever the weather permits. Homes literally require airing, and a fresh breeze on a nice day will usher out indoor air pollutants and bring new life and energy into your home.
- Regular cotton is one of the most pesticide-laden crops on the planet. Organic cotton is always a better choice, even if it costs a little more. Nobody needs to sleep in PJs made from fabrics that were ever doused in pesticides, created in a laboratory, or treated

Hemp: Not What You Thought

Hemp is an amazingly earth-friendly material, but some people avoid it because they believe it is somehow associated with, or is the same thing as, marijuana. However, hemp is not the same as marijuana. They are related, like distant cousins, but the hemp plant does not contain THC, the psychoactive substance in marijuana. It's simply an incredibly sturdy and hearty plant that makes excellent fabric. (The oil and seeds from the hemp plant are also excellent sources of essential fatty acid, with a delicious nutty taste—and no drug effect!)

Because hemp is so renewable and vigorous, it doesn't require pesticides or fertilizers, so hemp fabric is likely to be nontoxic. It's also durable, beautiful, and gets softer every time you wash it.

with toxic chemical dyes. Dress your family in organic cotton or hemp pajamas dyed with natural plant dyes. They're easier to find than you may think! Before I left working with Tom and Anne's family, I bought them all matching organic PJs for Christmas, which I found at Target.

Tom and Anne wasted no time making the changes I suggested, and when Baby Tommy arrived, their home was clean, pure, and ready for anything Tommy could dish out.

I recognize that all together, these changes can be expensive. Detoxing your home is the same as detoxing your body. If you can't do it all at once, do it step by step, gradually. When a room needs to be painted, get a nontoxic paint, but in the meantime, don't worry about paint that still looks fine.

If you need a new mattress, get an organic one. The same goes for bedding and clothing. Remember: Use it up, then upgrade it, and if appropriate (in the case of chemical cleaners or garden pesticides and fertilizers, for example), phase them out. Step by step, little by little, you will detox and purify your home and everything in it.

Be a Greener Cleaner

The next thing I want you to know about is cleaning products. Of course you want a clean home! A clean home is a peaceful home, but some ways of cleaning come at a price. If you use chemical cleaners and spray every surface with germ killers, you may be living in a very clean chemical soup.

The way you clean your home can have a significant impact on the cleanliness of your indoor air and the toxic nature of your carpets and floors. It can also affect the planet, because where does that phosphate-filled dishwasher soap go? What about that noxious toilet bowl cleaner, and those chemicals you spray to clean your sinks and counters? It all goes right down your drain—and straight into the water supply.

But you can be a greener cleaner. The first step is to switch from chemical cleaners that most people use to chemical-free, biodegradable cleaners. Use up the cleaners you have (you might as well because if you don't, you'll have to dispose of them somehow), but when they are gone, replace the all-purpose cleaners, glass cleaners, dishwashing soap, toilet-bowl cleaner, scouring powder, floor cleaner, and laundry detergent with upgraded versions. You'll be keeping chemicals in them out of the

---

Beware of Greenwashing

Don't be fooled by a green bottle or a picture of a plant on a cleaning product—instead, read the label to see what is really in that cleaner. The cleaner should contain only natural plant extracts, not chemicals. Some cleaners slightly reduce the chemicals or leave one chemical out but keep the rest, or add plant extracts to the chemicals, and they still call themselves "green." This is called greenwashing. A few brands I like and trust are:

- Mrs. Meyer's
- Seventh Generation
- Method
- Simple Green

groundwater, as well as out of your home. Many brands are widely available now, so check your local supermarket.

Or, to save more money, go back to basics. You probably have everything you need to clean anything in your home, right in your own kitchen. This simple, chemical-free, homemade, all-purpose cleaner is good for kitchen and bathroom counters, sinks, even toilets and bathtubs. Put it in a spray bottle and label it so you remember what it is: Organic Nanny Cleaner!

Here's how to make it:

Organic Nanny Cleaner
1. In a clean spray bottle, put 1 teaspoon of Castile soap, or other soap made with vegetable oils (conventional soap is made from animal fat).
2. Add 1 tablespoon of white vinegar.
3. Add 10 drops of lavender essential oil or tea tree oil.
4. Fill up the rest of the bottle with warm water. Cap tightly.

Use this cleaner to spray on counters, sinks, and floors. Just wipe or mop clean.

Other household products do a good job of cleaning, too. Try these:

- Here's a revelation: hot water and a little soap actually clean most things that get dirty, from walls and floors to counters and fixtures. Obvious, right? (Use soap made with vegetable oil, such as Castile soap.)
- Vinegar is a miracle substance! It's good on your salad greens, and it dissolves soap scum and hard water buildup. That's because it's an acid, but not the kind that will eat through your plumbing or your skin. Vinegar doesn't need a skull and crossbones or big hazard warnings on its label.
- Baking soda deodorizes and makes a great cleansing scrub for sinks and tubs. Sprinkle it on, mix with a bit of water, and scrub. Pour one cup down your drain and follow it with one cup of white vine-

Slow Death by Rubber Duck

Mamas, I hope you will check out this important book: *Slow Death by Rubber Duck: The Secret Danger of Everyday Things* by Rick Smith and Bruce Lourie. It goes into great depth to demonstrate how children are most at risk from the many chemicals in our environment, and explains the many serious ailments linked to toxic chemicals. The authors argue that environmental issues and health issues are the same issues, and that the health of our children is the greatest and most urgent environmental issue of our time. One reviewer wrote, "If readers don't change their ways after reading this one, then they never will."

gar for a fun, fizzy science experiment that also clears your drain of gunk and stink.

- Use plant oil. Linseed oil cleans and polishes wood (find it in your home improvement store). Essential oils such as lavender and tea tree oil have natural antibacterial properties, and add a nice smell to your homemade cleaners (find them at natural foods stores).

Detox the Bathroom

Little Bea, named after Beatrix Potter, was an adorable, red-headed three-year-old who loved to see her name on the Peter Rabbit books and had two bunnies as pets. She was the most trusting and easy-going little girl I ever met, and spoke with a cute British accent, just like her mother. She also loved bathtime, mostly because of her collection of bubble bath and shampoo bottles shaped and designed like many of her favorite characters from children's shows and toys—Big Bird, Elmo, Barbie.

But Bea also had a problem—chronic urinary tract infections. She used to tell me, "Nanny, it hurts to pee!" I watched her carefully to determine what could be causing this imbalance. The doctors didn't know—they just sent her poor distraught mother home with prescription after prescription. Then, I just happened to read something that mentioned commercial bubble bath was often the cause of cystitis in children, a painful irritation of the urethra.

I eyed those cute little bottles of bubble bath with suspicion—then emptied them, rinsed them clean, and filled them back up with organic bath soap and shampoo made for children. I refilled the bottles, so she wouldn't miss her "friends."

Sensitive Bea noticed immediately—no chemical perfume smell during bathtime, just the faint, pleasant scent of lavender and citrus. "This smells like oranges and flowers!" she exclaimed.

Because she was a smart little girl, I explained to her that the old soap had yucky things in it, but that this new soap was gentle and would keep her clean without hurting her. I'll never forget what she said because it represents how seriously children take marketing and advertising. She said: "But Big Bird and Elmo are my friends—they would never hurt me!" Then she turned and pointed her cute little soapy hand at Big Bird and said, "There will be no more of that, Mister Big Bird, or you will be in big trouble!"

I pointed at Bea's brother's bottles of Batman bubble bath and shampoo and told them, "You guys are next!"

Perhaps I don't need to tell you that she never had another urinary tract infection.

If you are going to bathe your children or yourself in something, or put something on any human skin, be sure it's pure! Skin is permeable. It breathes, which means it can take in anything it touches. Look for organic personal hygiene products that don't contain any of the following:

- Artificial fragrances, dyes (colors), and alcohol
- BHA
- Boric acid and its derivatives (like e.g., sodium borate)
- Bronopol
- DMDM hydantoin
- Oxybenzone
- Parabens
- Phthalates

Organic Nanny Notes

According to a report called "No More Toxic Tub" by the Campaign for Safe Cosmetics (CSC), dozens of popular bath products marketed for children contain the cancer-causing chemicals formaldehyde and 1,4-dioxane. Out of twenty-eight products tested for formaldehyde and forty-eight products tested for 1,4-dioxane, 61 percent contained both ingredients, 82 percent contained formaldehyde, and 67 percent contained 1,4-dioxane.

Even small exposures add up, especially if more than one product is used on a child or infant, says the CSC. They aren't disclosed on product labels because they are contaminants, not purposefully added ingredients.

According to the CSC, these ingredients, while banned in other countries, are not currently regulated in the United States. To avoid them, avoid common ingredients likely to be contaminated with:

- Quaternium-15
- Diazolidinyl urea
- DMDM hydantoin
- Imidazolidinyl urea

To find the actual report and complete list of tested products and the results, go to safecosmetics.org. To find products likely to be safer by choosing those with a short list of recognizable ingredients, check out the Environmental Working Group's Skin Deep Cosmetic Safety Database at www.cosmeticsdatabase.com.

- Sulfates (e.g., sodium lauryl sulfate and ammonium laureth sulfate)
- Triclosan

Planetary Prescription

Detoxing your home is crucial, but just as crucial, I would argue, is to keep in mind your larger home—your community, your state, your country, and your planet. I talked about environmental consciousness in Chapter 6, but I think it's relevant here as well because the condition of the Earth's air, water, soil, and wildlife matters. It impacts your health, your child's health, and the health of humans in general. Do we really want to put an end to ourselves through foolishness and wastefulness, greed and carelessness? Do we really want to trash our global home?

Instead, let's detox it! When your family does its part to keep your environment clean, and when you vote for those lawmakers who are doing their part on a larger scale, and when you teach your children to care for the natural world, change will happen. Your children will inherit a cleaner world than the one you inherited, not a more toxic one. Then, they can take over the stewardship of the Earth responsibly and compassionately.

Here are some more easy ways to make a difference:

- Recycle. Fill up that curbside box or just take those plastics, paper, and cans to the recycling center once a week. Make it a family affair, so your kids can help and you can answer questions about why you are bothering. Like: "The planet is filled up with trash—there isn't much more room, so we are going to make less!"
- Reuse or buy used items instead of buying new things all the time. The less new stuff you buy, the less you will throw away.
- When you must buy new, buy things with minimal packaging, preferably recyclable.
- Turn off lights, computers, and televisions when you aren't using them. Turn off the water if you are just standing there brushing your teeth. Don't turn on the shower until you really are ready to get in. Don't let the sink faucet run while you aren't actually rinsing a dish or a vegetable.
- Drive less. Take the bus, ride your bike, or just walk, if possible. You'll get more exercise and you'll keep the air cleaner.
- Buy from environmentally responsible companies. Ask questions. Vote with your dollars to send the message that you care about the fate of our planet.

- Bring your canvas bags to the grocery store. If you forget and must choose paper or plastic, choose paper.
- Drink your water from a stainless-steel water bottle instead of a plastic one. (All the cool yoga moms have stainless-steel bottles these days!)
- Bring your ceramic or covered travel mug with you to the coffee shop and fill it up instead of using paper or Styrofoam.
- Do you really need the ATM receipt? If not, hit the "no receipt" button.
- Don't use lawn chemicals where your children and pets play! Many lawn care companies now offer organic options.

And if you sometimes get tired of trying, tired of recycling or reusing, tired of conservation and vigilance, or if your children sometimes ask, "Why do we have to recycle/reuse/conserve/care?" then remind them, and yourself, how you feel. Remind them of L.O.V.E.

Explain what L.O.V.E. means.

Tell them that when you care about your family, then you begin to care about your community, which nurtures your family, and then you begin to care about your country, which nurtures your community, and then you begin to care about your whole world.

> *Organic Voices*
>
> Take nothing but pictures,
> leave nothing but footprints,
> kill nothing but time.
>
> —*John Kay*

Love expands. The boundaries of your caring just keep getting larger and larger until you realize that if you don't care for and nurture and take care of your own home, by which I mean our beautiful blue and green planet, then you will have nowhere left to go—no world, no country, no community, no family.

We are all connected, at every level, one to the other: children to parents to friends to all living breathing beings, and all of us to water, to air, to earth. This is why we must take care. Children who learn this become the people who can lead us into a future that will be better, not worse; more alive, not less.

Organic Nanny To-Do List

☐ Switch at least one chemical cleaning product to an organic one.

☐ Start phasing out carpets, curtains, bedding, and even clothing made of artificial materials.

☐ The next time you have to paint, find a nontoxic paint with no volatile organic compounds (VOCs). Look for paint labeled "non-VOC" or "no VOCs."

☐ Replace your child's bath products with organic versions.

☐ Do two environmentally conscious things this week that you wouldn't normally do, such as recycling and choosing a product with less packaging.

CHAPTER NINE

Phenomenal Mama Makeover

'Cause I'm a woman
Phenomenally.
Phenomenal woman,
That's me.

—Maya Angelou

Kristiane was a beautiful mama I worked with a few years ago. She had six-year-old twin girls and a three-year-old little boy, and she put enormous pressure on herself to do everything right. She cooked dinner almost every night. She found clever ways to get her children to eat fruit and vegetables (she even taught me a few tricks!). Her children were sweet and mostly well behaved, and always well dressed, with combed hair and clean hands. Kristiane volunteered at her daughters' school, worked part time at a hospital, and kept a spotless house. Her husband, a busy lawyer, was proud of her and her friends often commented that they didn't know how she could do it all.

But I saw another side to Kristiane when I came to help her with her children. She had dark circles under her eyes. She was low on energy but would push herself to extremes to get everything done, even if it meant staying up past midnight to clean up the clutter. She never took any time for herself because she was always so busy doing things for other people, and I could see the toll life was taking on her.

I'm a nanny for children, it's true. However, I often think of myself as a nanny for families, not just children, and who is the real head of the family on the home front? Of course, it is the mamas. Everyone goes to the mother first. If it's about the children, the home, the food, the cleaning, even the pets, it's always, "Ask Mom." When I first approached Kristiane about what I saw, I wanted to be gentle about it. One afternoon when the children were all down for a nap and she had just come home from work, I put my hand on her shoulder and I said, "How are *you* feeling?" When I said that to her, she looked at me for a moment, startled, and then burst into tears.

I've worked with so many mothers whom I've witnessed running themselves ragged. You spend so much of your time and energy giving, giving, giving your love and care away to your family and friends. It's one of the qualities that makes you so beautiful and valuable and beloved. But if you aren't also caring for yourself, it could all slip away. You won't enjoy your life as much. You won't be there for your children if you can't be there for yourself. As you let stress and neglect get the better of your body, mind, and spirit, the calm, centered, lovely woman you are at your core can begin to fray at the edges and fall apart.

> ### Organic Voices
>
> Every thought has the power to bring into being the visible from the invisible. It is absolutely necessary for us all to understand that everything we think, do or say comes back to us. Every thought, word or action—without exception—manifests itself as an actual reality.
>
> —*Ann Wigmore*

My dream for you is that you can be that mother you really want to be; and the wife you want to be; and the friend, and the helper, even the organic revolutionary, if that's what you want to be—but still be someone who knows who she is and takes some time each day to be quiet with herself and regain her inner calm and composure. Mamas, you need this time and you need to take care of yourselves. Otherwise, you won't be any good to anyone. This is so important! You are the key. You hold the household together, and as you go, so goes the family. So why are you going down the drain?

For many mothers, I believe the lack of self-care has become almost an emergency situation. It's you-time, and it's long overdue.

It's time to dig deep inside your soul and pull out the weeds to make room for the seeds of vibrant health and happiness. This isn't so hard, Mamas. The weeds are your bad health habits and your self-neglect, but the flowers you'll grow when you cultivate your own inner soil will be so beautiful that you'll wonder why you ever forgot to water them.

In this chapter, then, I'd like to focus on *you*. How would you like to have:

- More energy
- Vibrant skin
- Sound sleep
- A healthy body at a healthy weight
- Less stress and anxiety
- More peace and happiness

That sounds good to me, too. Are you ready for a Phenomenal Mama Makeover?

Six Steps to Reclaiming Fabulous

I believe that finding your way back to yourself is not all that hard and not all that time consuming. The problem is, mothers just don't often make it a priority. I'd like to show you how to do it by trying just six easy things:

1. Prioritizing whole foods
2. Reserving Sunday for Spa Day
3. Learning how to meditate
4. Moving more
5. Nurturing your spirit
6. Connecting with your friends

These six simple tweaks can change your life. I asked Kristiane to try them, and she especially loved meditation. It was just the centering she needed. Other moms I've worked with have particularly embraced whole foods, or the idea of a Spa Sunday, or more time with friends, but I encourage all my mamas to try to incorporate all six changes into their lives. Maybe you already do some of them, but all of them are important, and none of them are difficult. They don't take too much time, and they really will make you a calmer, happier, more centered, more energized mom. Let's look at how to make each one happen for you.

1. Your New Obsession: Whole Plant Foods

The first, best, most important, most crucial thing an Organic Mama can do to nourish and boost her own health and energy is to eat whole plant foods. Out with the junk food, the fast food, the processed food! Just get it out. It's not doing you any favors, and the temporary comfort you think it provides is just a trick of addiction.

Whole plant foods have everything you need to be a healthy, happy mother with energy and love to spare: protein, complex carbohydrates, fiber, vitamins, minerals, and thousands of phytochemicals that tweak and refine your glowing health. Plus, on a plant-based diet, you'll feel lighter, airier, more optimistic. Things will seem brighter. You won't feel weighed down and heavy.

If you've read the book up to this point, you already know what I mean by whole plant foods. I mean L.O.V.E. foods. Local, Organic, Vegcentric or Vegetarian or Vegan, and Environmental. Some of the biggest energy destroyers are processed sugar (including high-fructose corn syrup and white sugar), fake fats (trans fats), and heavy animal foods such as meat, cheese, milk, and eggs. If you want to feel like you could dance through your day, focus your diet on plant foods. Bonus points: You're setting a great example for your kids! You can't expect them to love plant foods if you don't embrace them with everything you've got.

You don't need an Organic Nanny to tell you that junky processed food saps your energy and drains the glow from your cheeks. Instead, eat with L.O.V.E. to enliven your spirit and refresh your body, cleaning out

Hydration Miracle

Water is just as important for you as it is for your kids. Drink it all day long. Plastic bottles are an environmental hazard and some might even be toxic for you and your children, so refill a stainless-steel water bottle via a Brita filter or other water filtration system in your home, for the purest possible H_2O experience. Aim for at least 48 ounces, preferably more like 60 ounces each day. Herbal tea counts! When you stay well hydrated, your body works better, your skin looks better, you won't be so chronically hungry, and you'll have more energy. Sure, you may have to hover near a bathroom for a day or two until your body adjusts, but it will. Drink up! Consider it your power beauty secret.

the toxic gunk, and building strong, vibrant health. You'll grow slowly stronger and brighter and more energetic, and you'll nurture and tend the spark it takes to be an even better mom.

I've heard hundreds of stories from my clients with a long list of different health problems (chronic fatigue syndrome, fibromyalgia, arthritis, even heart disease) who experienced improvement and, in some cases, healing, simply by turning to clean whole foods: vegetables, fruits, legumes, whole grains, and nuts. I'm certainly not a doctor, but I don't think it takes a medical degree to know that this is good food that will boost your health. It's common sense and it's intuitive. When you get the junk and heavy foods out of your life for good, your life will absolutely transform. It sounds so simple, but it really works.

Reality Check

Of course, you may be thinking, "But Organic Nanny, it's easy for you to say I should switch to whole foods, but it isn't simple when I just can't keep my hands out of the chip bag or my purse where I keep my change that I use in the vending machine at work! And what about that invisible force that makes my car go through the drive-through?"

Oh, but Mamas, I *do* get it! You are addicted to the bad stuff, and I know how it feels because I've been there, too. I don't expect anything more or less of you than you expect of your children. That's why all the helpful hints in the first part of this book apply to you. You don't have to change all your bad habits at once. Start gradually. Begin by introducing more beautiful plant foods, and just see how you feel. Phase out the bad stuff from your life, whether it's chips or cookies or double lattes or that insidious vending machine. Go slowly. The more often you decide to eat fruit instead of candy, or a bowl of brown rice instead of a hunk of white bread with butter; or just to get out and breathe the fresh air and go on a walk instead of eating when you know you aren't really hungry, the better you will feel, and gradually, slowly but surely, those bad habits will lose their grip on your life.

I believe a lot of mothers eat poorly in search of instant comfort, but the long-term comfort, the feel-good feelings that really last, don't come from a candy bar or a cupcake (delicious as those might be in the moment). They come from taking care of yourself in the same way you would your own child. You are worthy of your own love and nurture, and I see how beautiful and sensitive you really are. Look in the mirror and find it for yourself, and then just start taking those baby steps. Pack as much whole plant foods into your day as you can, and soon you will find that there begins to be less room for the stuff that makes you feel good for a few minutes and bad for the rest of the day.

One thing that can happen when you give up your addictions is that you might notice a swelling up of emotions, both good and bad. You might get surges of joy or shadows of despair. This is just your body adjusting to a healthier diet. I always recommend that people sit with their feelings, whenever they feel that panicky urge to grab for food. Usually, this kind of feeling isn't about food. You've got plenty of food. There is no shortage. You will not starve. Sit, breathe, and think about what you are really hungry for. I bet it's not those neon-colored taco chips. I bet it's for something else.

Maybe you need a hug from your child or your husband or your friend. Maybe you just need to talk to somebody. Maybe you need to move that body of yours—shake it up, get outside, turn your face to the sun, breathe the fresh air. Maybe you need to pet your dog or cat, or just

---

Ask for Help

Changing your lifestyle can be challenging and stressful. Losing weight can seem impossible sometimes, and even painful, because when you don't let yourself eat for comfort, then you have to feel all those feelings you were trying to bury under a pile of food.

Never forget that you have help! Tata always used to say, "I ask God for help, and he sends me people." I told Kristiane, the mama who asked me for help, that this is why I came to her: to help. No matter what your spiritual beliefs, send out your request for help, and be open to answers. You never know who might step forward with answers. Two books I highly recommend to help with emotional eating: *Women, Food, and God* by Geneen Roth and *You Can Heal Your Life* by Louise L. Hay.

---

take a bath. Maybe you need to relax. Or maybe you're just trying to put off something that really needs doing.

Listen to yourself. Don't hold your ears and shut your eyes and yell, "Not listening, la la la la la!" at the feelings. Pay attention to them instead. Maybe they aren't as bad as you thought they were. Or maybe they are, but better to get them out of you than let them sit inside festering and urging you to eat another brownie. If you can take better care of yourself and learn to listen to your own heart, I bet you'll discover that most of those urges don't have anything at all to do with food.

Eating Is Okay!

And if you are taking care of yourself and you really are still hungry—don't deprive yourself. Sometimes it takes a while to get used to eating a new way, and you may find you eat a little bit more at first, and then a little bit less as time goes on and your body adjusts to the taste and nutrition in real, whole foods.

Feeling full from plant foods is a different kind of feeling than feeling full from animal products or junk foods. It's a lighter, calmer kind of fullness, rather than a heavy, comatose kind of fullness. You probably won't need a nap, but you might want to take a walk. Either way, this new kind of fullness is something you will learn to appreciate. It's very, very satisfying.

Another great thing about eating whole plant foods is that you never have to feel guilty about eating! You can fill up your plate with fresh raw salad, whole grains such as brown rice and couscous, and delicious veggie-based stews, sauces, and stir-fries. As long as your choices are whole grain, plant-derived, and low in fat, you really can't eat too much. You won't need to. The fiber in whole plant foods fills you up, and with a few strategic spices and herbs, the flavors will thrill you.

Here is an example of a day of eating whole L.O.V.E. foods—you can lose weight eating like this, and it might even be too much food for you! The better you nourish your body, the less will have to keep crying out for *more, more, more*!

Breakfast	Snack	Lunch	Snack	Dinner	Snack
Fruit smoothie filled with berries, a few leafy greens, and plant-based protein powder in the summer, or oatmeal with cinnamon, raisins, walnuts, and soy or almond milk in the winter; green tea or one cup of coffee (or try to work your way back down to one cup of coffee, if you can—no pressure)	Herbal tea and sliced pear or apple with sprinkle of walnuts or a little almond butter	Quinoa or brown rice pilaf with sautéed vegetables and black beans or chickpeas; small green salad with halved cherry tomatoes and a drizzle of sesame vinaigrette	Celery and carrot sticks with hummus	Black bean or other veggie burger on whole-grain bun, baked sweet potato fries, big green salad with your favorite chopped or steamed veggies and creamy vegan dressing (one of my favorites is Annie's Organic Goddess Dressing)	Baked tortilla chips with fresh avocados mashed with tomatoes; chamomile tea

You can model every meal after this plan, or get a great vegan cookbook and go crazy with delightful plant food cooking experiments. All you have to do is keep it all about the plants, and about the whole food. Focus on fruit and tea in the morning, and move toward vegetables, grains, and beans later in the day, with plenty of water along the way, and between each meal. A glass of organic wine with dinner is a nice addition, too. (Just keep it to one—more than one a day for women has been linked with increased cancer risk, but one can be healthful if you enjoy it.)

When the foods you choose are L.O.V.E. foods, you don't have to worry much about portion control. They will fill you up and make you feel great. Your body will reset, and it will even find its natural healthy weight. All you have to do is keep the good food coming in to keep the good feelings coming out.

2. Your New Mission: Spa Sundays

Don't you wish you could spend every Sunday at the spa? You could get a massage, maybe a salt scrub, take a relaxing yoga class, meditate, then maybe a mud bath, spend some time in the Jacuzzi, and a mani-pedi . . . Oh, but you can!

I propose that your new mission—well, one of them at least—is to make Sunday a day for *you*. Make it a day of pampering, of quiet, of mama time, and of purity. And by purity, I mean cleansing.

People have a lot of differing ideas about cleansing, but I believe that a weekly raw-food cleanse is one of the purest, sweetest things you can do for your own health. Cleansing works because it gives your digestive system a rest from dead processed food. I've always found Sunday to be a perfect day for a good cleanse.

Even if you don't consider Sunday a particularly holy day, it is often a day of relaxation, so it is well suited for a day of reduced food intake. However, I don't recommend strict fasting for mamas, who have to take care of their children (and everyone else). You need energy from real food.

That's why I suggest that every Sunday, you eat nothing but pure raw plant foods—freshly squeezed juice, juicy raw fruit, and crisp raw vegetables. Raw plant foods contain pure live enzymes, so they bring your

Anti-Cranky-Mama Snacks

You know that feeling when you just want to scream or pound on a pillow or give yourself a time-out in your room that lasts for, oh, I don't know, four or five hours? We all experience this, especially during PMS or when we haven't had enough sleep or haven't been eating well, or life just gets to be too much. Mothers are only human!

Fortunately, food can help calm the savage breast. The best way to fight that fatigue and crankiness is with an Organic Nanny–approved Anti-Cranky-Mama snack, when breakfast or lunch or dinner just weren't enough to get you to your happy place:

- A smoothie made by blending 1 cup of fresh or frozen fruit (e.g., frozen berries or a frozen banana), 1 handful of leafy greens (e.g., spinach or chopped kale), 1 cup of rice or soy milk, and a pinch of cinnamon. For extra richness or energy, add a spoonful of nut butter, a teaspoon of cocoa powder or raw cacao nibs, and/or a teaspoon of instant coffee or espresso powder.
- Sprouted grain toast (I like Ezekiel bread) with hummus, mashed white beans, or one-quarter of an avocado, sliced, with a sprinkle of sea salt
- A shot of wheatgrass from a juice bar (on an empty stomach). (Warning: This is intense and some people really hate the taste. For those of us who like it or who can get used to it, however, it immediately turns the whole day around!)
- Fresh apple slices with natural (no sugar added) peanut butter or almond butter
- A bunch of fresh grapes and a small handful of raw walnuts
- AB&J (like PB&J for grown-ups): sprouted grain toast with almond butter and no-sugar fruit spread
- If you feel you absolutely must eat something from a package, let it be a Larabar (dried fruit and nuts, all raw, no sugar, but you'd never know it) or a Rice Dream Pie (cookies and ice cream dipped in chocolate, but made entirely from brown rice, with no cane sugar or dairy—mmm!).

body back to life. Drink plenty of water to wash out the toxins as your body goes into self-cleaning mode, and have an easy day. If you need warmth, drink a comforting cup of herbal or green tea. I like to brew a big pot of mint tea in the morning and sip on it all day. It will help settle your stomach.

If this doesn't work for you because you are a big-Sunday-dinner kind of family, then just do raw food up until dinner. This will help your body clean out and calm down and get ready to adjust to a bigger meal.

But your day of purity is about more than food. It's about cleansing and calming in every possible way. You may still be busy, you may still have things you have to do, but try to squeeze in as many spa-like activities as you possibly can. Ask your family to give you just a little bit of time to yourself, and use it wisely. Take a long bath. Scrub your skin with a brush, or one of the homemade scrubs I'll tell you about. Give yourself a long and thorough mani-pedi, complete with foot soak and nail polish. Curl up with a book or your favorite old movie that you never watch because nobody else ever wants to see it again. Take a walk in nature somewhere, by yourself or not. Breathe deeply. Meditate. Take a nap. Pray. Or just hug your family and hang out with them for a while without actually *doing anything.*

It's a beautiful feeling to take time for yourself, and when it becomes a habit, Spa Sundays will bring peace, joy, and purity into your life every day of the week. And you won't believe how great food will taste on Monday. It's like pressing the reset button on your body. It's like being born again.

Here are some more ideas for pampering yourself the Organic Nanny way.

Organic Mama Sunday Spa Treatments

Don't spend hundreds of dollars on fancy spa treatments. Instead, make them at home from your own simple, pure, natural, organic ingredients. Especially indulge in the scrubs, which help get toxins out of your skin as your body purges them during your raw food cleanse. All these scrubs can be stored in an airtight container (like a glass jar with a lid) in the refrigerator.

Sea Salt Scrub

Mix 1 cup of sea salt and 1 cup of almond oil with 5 drops of lavender essential oil (or other essential oil you like, such as orange, almond, or mint). Stir together, then scoop up and gently rub on your skin. Shower off.

Cuban Sugar Scrub

Combine 1 cup of white or brown sugar, 1/4 cup of orange juice, 1/4 cup of fresh mango puree, and 1/2 cup of coconut oil. Stir well. Smooth over skin. Let it sit for five minutes, then shower off. The sugar and fruit acids slough off dead skin and the coconut oil softens rough patches. You'll feel silky-smooth and gorgeous.

Organic Nanny Massage Oil

When you're feeling tense, stir up a batch of this yummy massage oil. Touch alone has demonstrated pain-relieving benefits, and this oil will make you feel even better. Rub it on yourself, or better yet, have someone else do it for you. Your husband can rub your shoulders and back with it, or gently rub it on your belly when you have menstrual cramps or just feel bloated and cranky from PMS. (One week a month, I call this "PMS Oil.")

This makes a great all-over massage oil, as well as a gentle face and body oil to soothe dry skin: Combine 1 cup of almond oil, the contents of one vitamin E capsule (snip it open and squeeze it in), 5 drops of lavender essential oil, and 5 drops of ylang-ylang or orange essential oil. Stir gently and pour into a pretty antique jar or old perfume bottle. Bottles of this lovely oil also make great gifts—100 percent handmade, no animal testing.

If you're not quite up to making your own beauty products, that doesn't mean you can't have just as luxurious of a spa day. I suggest you splurge just a little on natural spa and cosmetic products that are vegan, and by that I mean they were not tested on animals. Products may or may not say so on the label—call the company if you aren't sure.

To make your selection easier, just check out the cosmetics counter at your local health food and beauty store, or look for cruelty-free cosmetics and beauty products online. Many companies are well known for their commitment to animal-friendly products and their stance against animal testing. Some produce only products without any animal-derived ingredients. For a complete and comprehensive list, see PETA's Web site at www.mediapeta.com/peta/PDF/companiesdonttest.pdf.

3. Your New Contemplation: Morning Meditation

Maybe it sounds boring or impossible, but meditation is just about the easiest—and hardest—thing you can do that will make a huge impact on your life. Really, it's just a way to calm your mind, center yourself, and breathe. It's like a reset button, and it's also kind of like weightlifting for your brain. Meditation makes your brain stronger.

I believe meditation is a crucial practice for anyone dealing with stress. It isn't technically difficult and there are many ways to do it. You might not like one way, but you might love another. Start with just five minutes each morning. Meditation will start your day out on just the right note.

Meditation looks easy. You're just sitting there, for Pete's sake! However, it can be challenging and even frustrating at first, if you have one of those brains that never stops chattering. Don't let that deter you, Mamas—you need meditation more than you know! The beauty of this simple practice is that it gets easier, and fast. The more you do it on a regular schedule, the calmer you'll feel and the more you will enjoy a sense of control over your formerly wayward brain.

How to do it? That's the easy part. Set the alarm for just five or ten minute earlier. Get up and immediately sit back down. Ahhh. Sit comfortably, close your eyes, and think of one word, such as *heal* or *love* or *heart* or *peace*. Repeat it in your mind, over and over. When your mind wanders away from the word (which it will), just notice this and go back to the word. Five minutes and done!

Another technique is to focus on your breath. Feel it moving in and out of your body. Listen to its sound. Is it cold or warm in your nose or throat? Is it quick or slow? Follow it without trying to control it. When your mind wanders, gently bring it back. Visualizing is also a way to relax and relieve stress. Visualize the day ahead going perfectly in your mind's eye. Thoughts can create your reality, so when you make an effort to think positively, you are more likely to feel positive. Visualizing is also fun. Imagine walking the beach or strolling through the woods or a field of flowers. Instant relaxation!

Another technique is to just be quiet inside and listen and feel the world around you. Just be, in the present moment, and when your mind wanders to the past or future or anything else that isn't actually going on around you, gently bring it back to the now, as if it is a little wandering toddler whom you guide gently back to her carpet square. Music can help make this easier because it gives you something very specific to focus on. Use meditation music (you can purchase this kind of music online and transfer it to your iPod or other media player). Daily affirmations are yet another cool form of meditation. I had one mama client, Cindy, who could not get her thoughts focused. Daily affirmation meditation helped her tremendously. She liked to say, "I am healthy and strong," on some days, and on other days, she would say, "My children live in my heart."

Here are some positive affirmations you can try, or make up something similar that is important to you. Sit comfortably, breathe, and then repeat ten times, aloud and in your mind:

I love and am loved.
My body is strong and beautiful.
We are all one.
I am doing all the right things to have an amazing life.
My life is exceptional. I am exceptional.
I feed my body healthy foods.
Today I will achieve my dreams.
I have everything I need.
What I think is what I am.
My actions create my reality.

Now, try to visualize what you are saying as you say it. See the words being true and believe them. Remember, what you think about grows in your life.

Rather than skip meditation because you don't like it, find a way to do it that you love, and watch it change you. Meditation is so important, I wish everyone did it! I believe the world would be a more loving place. At least your home can be a more loving place. Meditate and love yourself and never be self-critical! You're the star of your own life. Now *that's* something to meditate on!

4. Your New Passion: Body in Motion

A healthier, calmer, stronger, more confident you requires one more step—movement. Now don't roll your eyes, Mama—exercise really is the closest thing to a miracle you will ever find when you are looking for ways to have more energy and feel better about yourself and your world. But exercise doesn't have to be what you think it is: boring and hard. It can be fun. Just as with meditation, all you have to do is find a way to exercise that you can live with. Walking? Yoga? A running club? The elliptical trainer at the gym with the personal television tuned to your favorite show? Hey, whatever it takes!

When I think about mamas and the importance of exercise, I remember Susan. Susan was a forty-year-old mom with four young daughters, and I was their nanny a few years ago. A former dancer for New York City Ballet, Susan had stopped being active several years before, as her "mom duties" increased. Yet, her fatigue seemed to outweigh even the heavy demands on her time. She was diagnosed with chronic fatigue syndrome and had what I considered to be a startling number of prescriptions to help her get through the day.

When the family called for my services, I came to meet them. Susan could barely function, and needed some help while she tried to regain her health. The problem was, she had no idea how to do it. After I settled in, she asked if she could speak with me one evening. We sat down, and I listened.

"I'm scared," she said. "I can barely move. I'm so tired in the mornings, I can't stand the thought of getting out of bed, and just look at me!" She gestured toward her own figure, her voice full of despair. "I'm getting fat!"

Susan used to be thin and strong, dancing six days a week before she had children, but it was clear to me that she had stopped caring for herself as she poured all her efforts into caring for them. And yet, ironically, she couldn't be there for them anymore because she was too worn down.

Organic Nanny Top Three Favorite Energy Tips

1. *Wheatgrass.* Wheatgrass juice is one of nature's true superfoods. Just 2 ounces of juice provides the same nourishment as up to 4 pounds of fresh, green vegetables! It's energizing and can help your body combat increased stress or illness. The chlorophyll in wheatgrass also helps to purify the liver, and wheatgrass can also be useful in treating constipation. You can buy a wheatgrass shot at a juice bar, or grow your own wheatgrass (some natural foods stores sell little pots of wheatgrass) and juice it at home yourself, although this requires a special kind of juicer. Some health food stores also sell frozen shots you can defrost and drink at home. Just to warn you, wheatgrass has an intense taste, and not everyone can take it. But wow, talk about an energy boost! The more you drink it, the more you will learn to love what it can do for you.

2. *Sunshine.* Take a walk on a sunny day, or just step outside and feel the sun on your face and arms for about ten minutes. Sunshine generates vitamin D production and lifts your spirits. It also fills you up with energy. Take deep breaths of fresh air while you're out there. That helps, too.

3. *Vitamin B_{12}.* Many people, especially vegans, may be deficient in this important vitamin, but there are good ways to get your dose. Your doctor can give you a quick shot of the good stuff, but not everyone likes the idea of getting an injection. Another great way to get your B_{12} is through a spray that you spray under your tongue. This is much better absorbed than a B_{12} supplement in pill form. There is also evidence that B_{12} can significantly increase your metabolism, which can lead to very natural, easy weight loss, especially if you are B_{12} deficient. Ask your doctor whether a B_{12} supplement might be helpful for you.

"You're the Organic Nanny," she pleaded with me. "Can you help me? Is there some kind of diet you can recommend? I want to play with my kids again. I want to move. I want to feel alive again. What's your secret? What can I do? I need help. I know you're a nanny for the children, but I think I need one, too!"

Susan's husband stood by, grimly. He had been spending more and more of his time caring for the children because his wife just couldn't. This is why they hired me. She knew she was putting too much of a burden on him, and he wanted to help her, but I could tell the family was hanging by a thread. They needed help, and they needed it now.

My secret special "prescription" for Susan was to eat a whole-foods, plant-based diet and restart her exercise regimen. At first, she resisted. "I'm too tired to exercise!" she insisted. I asked if she was too tired for a stroll around the block after dinner in the evening. She hesitated, then admitted that maybe she could do that.

I set to work cooking whole-food meals for the family, showing Susan what I was doing and how I was doing it. That first night, after dinner, the family waited together in the living room, expectantly, as Susan walked around the block. She wanted to go alone, and I supported her. This woman needed some time to herself! When she returned, just fifteen minutes later, I could tell this was going to work. She had a flush back in her cheeks, and she was smiling. "I didn't go very fast," she told us proudly, but I made it! And I actually feel pretty good."

Walking became Susan's new "doctor," and along with her new diet that gave her more energy, pretty soon she began to alternate walking with jogging, and then running. After a while, she switched her exercise time to mornings.

It wasn't always smooth sailing. Sometimes, when life got extra busy or something stressful happened, Susan would lapse, or be tempted to skip a morning run. I began to put her running shoes right next to her bed every night, so she would see them as soon as she awoke. This usually worked, and Susan began to do it herself. When I left the family, Susan had lost 20 pounds, was regaining her muscle definition, and looked, at least to me, like a completely new woman.

Exercise gets the blood moving through your body, oxygenates your tissues and organs, and also activates your lymphatic system, which can become sluggish and congested if you spend most of your day sitting. The lymphatic system is like a vacuum cleaner for your immune system. Sweating and moving and using your muscles gets the lymph pumping, and then you really start to feel clean on the inside.

Sleep On It

Exercise is fantastic for you, but sleep is just as crucial to balance that exercise and give your body a chance to heal. Most mamas don't get enough sleep. If you feel tired during the day, make sleep a priority. It's more important than television, Mamas! Get yourself right on up to bed. If you have problems with sleeping, check out Chapter 9, where I give you some natural cures for insomnia.

Exercise can't cure every illness. It didn't erase Susan's chronic fatigue syndrome, but it certainly made her life easier, and it's likely to make anybody feel better than they felt without it, no matter what other physical condition they might have.

You can make the same kinds of changes happen for yourself, too. No matter what you are or are not doing, just start moving. It's mama maintenance!

As for what to do, exercise is what you make of it. Walking is excellent and almost anyone can do it, but there are so many other ways to fit physical activity into your day. Some types of exercise popular with mothers include:

- *Yoga.* There are many types of yoga, from sweaty Bikram-style hot yoga to dancelike Vinyasa yoga to precision alignment-oriented Iyengar yoga or heart-opening Anusara yoga. These are just a few popular styles, but there are many more. Yoga can be invigorating, energizing, relaxing, calming, and healing, or all of these in one class. I highly recommend it.
- *Pilates.* This core-strengthening exercise regimen has helped many women gain strength, improve posture, and get slimmer. It's fun and many gyms as well as Pilates studios offer classes or individual sessions.
- *Gym membership.* Some mothers love to go to the gym. It's their time they give to themselves. Gyms can be fun because they offer many

Rub It In

Another spectacular way to get your lymphatic system activated is massage. Massage works tension out of your muscles and gets everything moving along the way it should. It's also a great way to relax and de-stress. I advise all stressed-out mamas to get a massage at least once a month. Some massage therapists use essential oils with scents specifically designed to relax you. The use of essential oils for therapeutic reasons is called aromatherapy. It's the perfect complement to a massage. Or, swap massages with your husband, using the massage oil recipe in this chapter.

different kinds of exercise machines for cardio and weightlifting, plus such features as spinning classes (you ride an exercise bike while the instructor guides you through the "ride"), classes that combine weightlifting with music, step aerobics, kick boxing or other martial arts–inspired cardio classes, and many more. Many gyms also offer yoga and/or Pilates classes; may have swimming pools; and often have saunas, steam rooms, Jacuzzis, or showers, so you can go to the gym, clean up, and get ready for work all in one place.

- *Bicycling.* If you love the outdoors and you love to explore, try riding a bicycle each day, especially if you live in a bike-friendly city. Don't forget to wear your helmet!
- *Training for a 5K, half-marathon, triathalon, or marathon.* Having a goal can help mamas get moving. Many cities have regular races and you may also be able to find groups or clubs that train together. Or train on your own with your own regimen. You might surprise yourself!
- *Dance.* Whether you take a ballet, modern dance, belly-dancing, or hip-hop class, or something more fitness related such as Zumba, dance classes can be so much fun that they don't even feel like exercise. Many dance studios offer classes for adults. Don't be shy! Channel your inner ballerina, or be a hip-hop queen. Why shouldn't you have this much fun? Or, if you prefer getting a little racy, try a

My Top Four Energy Foods

1. *Avocados.* Use in sweet or savory dishes. Try them in cakes and pudding!
2. *Green lemonade juice.* Order this from the juice bar, or juice fresh lemons with a handful of leafy greens such as kale, stir in agave syrup, and pour over ice!
3. *Almond butter.* This is the grown-up answer to peanut butter!
4. *Coconut oil.* Smelling as good as it tastes, it's the perfect oil for sautéing veggies, and it's also great for dry skin!

pole-dancing class! These classes give you a great workout, burlesque style. They don't allow any men into the class, so you can let loose and not feel self-conscious.

These are just a few ideas. There are so many ways to move and use your muscles and get strong and conditioned. This is important, Mamas. This is your life, and when you are fit, you'll be in the best possible shape to really live it.

5. Your New Vision: Spirituality

There is another part of you that you must not neglect if you want to be a fulfilled and balanced mama: your spirit. Spirit is easy to neglect because you can't see it. It doesn't show up on the scale or in the mirror, but it's there nevertheless, and it requires just as much maintenance as your body and your mind. Please just take a few minutes every day to stop, breathe, center yourself, and think about who you are and where you are going. If you practice a particular religion, devote some time, thought, prayer, or contemplation to that. How does it feed you? Are there other ways you can become more involved? Can you bring more spirituality into your family? A 1998 study from the University of Michigan showed that high school seniors who said religion was important in their lives and who attended some kind of religious service regularly had lower rates of alcohol use, cigarette smoking, drug use, carrying weapons, and getting into fights. These students also had higher rates of seat belt use and consumed a healthier diet. Other studies have showed that people who consider themselves religious or spiritual, whether they actually belong to an organized religion or not, recover from illness more quickly and generally have better health habits.

I'm not saying you have to convert to some religion you don't believe in. What I am saying is that if you can become more aware of your spiritual side, think about what you believe, and have faith in those beliefs, you are likely to benefit. You are more than a mother, a wife, a homemaker, an employee. You are a unique spiritual being with a path and a purpose, and when you let yourself consider this and act on it, you are likely to be happier and healthier. What have you got to lose? Many of the mamas I know aren't particularly religious but they do believe in a higher power or a universe that guides events and listens to prayers and intentions. A fun way to tap into this connection is to make a vision board. A vision board is a collage that represents everything you consider a priority in your life, or a goal you want to reach, and you get to use scissors and glue sticks! You could invite your children to make their own vision boards with you, or make it a personal experience. It's a fun activity for a rainy day, but it's more than a one-time activity. It is a way to set your intentions purposefully. Here's how to do it:

Organic Voices

Whatever you vividly imagine, ardently desire, sincerely believe, and enthusiastically act upon … must inevitably come to pass!

–Paul J. Meyer

First, gather your supplies: A poster board from your local craft or art store, scissors, glue stick, and a pile of old magazines you no longer need.

Flip through photographs and magazines and cut out any pictures and words that represent the things you most value or the things you would like to have more of in your life. Some examples might be pictures of families spending time together, healthy children, healthy mothers, people who are fit and active, healthy foods, beautiful places you'd like to go someday, or pictures that represent more financial security. If the environment is important to you, look for beautiful natural scenes. If you want to improve your relationship with your husband, or you are looking for love in your life, include romantic pictures. If you want to be a better athlete, find pictures showing people running or doing yoga poses or whatever it is you would like to achieve. Find inspiring words that make you feel like your best self. It's up to you—whatever you want and need and love, include those things on your vision board. Whatever speaks to you and your desires and dreams, cut them out and include them in your picture.

Next, arrange your cut-outs on the poster board and glue them down with loving care. Put your vision board somewhere in your home where you will see it every day, but visitors might not necessarily see it (these visions are for you and you alone). Look at it, and really see it, every day. What you dream about, think about, and strive for will come to you, and this is a way to make those dreams more concrete and central in your vision.

About once a year, make a new vision board, as your dreams and desires evolve. I like to make one right at the end of December, to help reset my intention for the new year. What you dream, you can do, in some way, and with self-care and self-love, all your dreams really will start coming true. I've seen it happen to many, many families, and that's why I know it can happen to you and yours.

6. Your New Commitment: Girlfriends!

The last item on your nurtured mama to-do list is no less important than any of the others. How long has it been since you've had coffee or a night out with your friends? It's so easy for mamas to put this off or cancel or just stop making plans when life gets too busy, but nurturing your friendships with other women can be your lifeline. Spending time with your female friends actually reduces stress and makes you feel better about yourself. In fact, one UCLA study I recently read about says that women respond to stress with a particular cascade of brain chemicals that cause them to seek out and maintain female friendships. So cherish your girlfriends, Mamas! They can provide you with the kind of support that you just can't get from the men in your life, no matter how wonderful those men might be.

Talk to your family about how important this is to you. I'm not saying you should be going out every night. Of course not; your family needs you! However, a monthly girl's night out, or a weekly coffee or tea date with a friend, or the occasional mani-pedi with your BFFs, is not too much to ask of any family. This is important, and it will make you feel better about your life. Girlfriends put things back into perspective. They listen and they really care. Sometimes, they can see what you couldn't see on your own. They are invaluable.

You are not alone, and you are worth treasuring, and your girlfriends can tell you that in ways your family may not, even though they know it to be true. This is why you need them.

It Starts with You

Some of the mamas I've worked for haven't had too much trouble incorporating more self-care, once they get a nudge. However, many of them still resist, and I know why. They feel selfish! So let me end this chapter with a little Organic Nanny lecture.

Mamas, if you don't take care of yourself, how will your children ever learn how to take care of *themselves*? How can you keep a food out of your children's diet, but continue to eat it yourself? How can you tell children to go outside and play, but refuse to exercise or get outside yourself? Your daughters in particular look to you as a model. How can you teach your daughters that they should be good to themselves, learn how to calm their own mind, have hopes and dreams and visions, if you don't do any of those things for yourself? Children strive to be like their parents, whether they admit it or not. Toddlers imitate Mommy and Daddy;

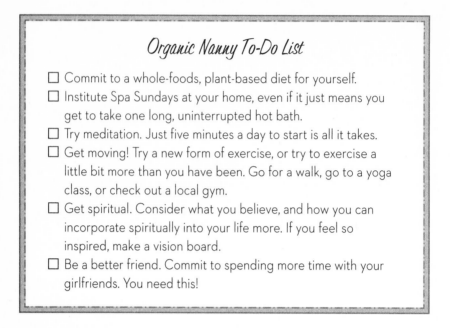

Organic Nanny To-Do List

- ☐ Commit to a whole-foods, plant-based diet for yourself.
- ☐ Institute Spa Sundays at your home, even if it just means you get to take one long, uninterrupted hot bath.
- ☐ Try meditation. Just five minutes a day to start is all it takes.
- ☐ Get moving! Try a new form of exercise, or try to exercise a little bit more than you have been. Go for a walk, go to a yoga class, or check out a local gym.
- ☐ Get spiritual. Consider what you believe, and how you can incorporate spiritually into your life more. If you feel so inspired, make a vision board.
- ☐ Be a better friend. Commit to spending more time with your girlfriends. You need this!

curious grade-schoolers navigating their own new sense of ethics will ask questions and look to you to learn what is right and wrong; teenagers may rebel, but then end up being more like their parents in the end than they ever thought they would be.

Tata always used to tell me: *"Empieza contigo!"* ("Start with yourself!") Mamas, this is so important. Start with yourself, and your family will follow, especially if you are instituting changes that might be difficult or encouraging behaviors that don't come naturally in our society, such as vegetarianism or no sugar or nightly family dinners or a sense of self-confidence and purpose in life, or a commitment to living in sync with nature. If you send your children down that road less traveled, you have to lead.

I can't count how many times I've told my clients to teach their children by example; then we'd walk together to the kitchen and start deciding which foods are going to get the old heave-ho. Often, it's the mothers who are objecting to putting those cookies into the trash, more than the kids! It's the mothers who suddenly "don't have time" to go on a bike ride, or sit for five minutes in meditation, or contemplate what's really important to them. Because they have to do what? Clean the bathroom? Do the laundry? Because *Dancing with the Stars* is on?

Mothers and fathers are often surprised at their children's ability to adapt to something new, especially if the whole family is doing it together. Children are naturally curious, and many pride themselves on standing out. If you make a game out of making better dietary choices, your children will want to play. If you commit to outdoor exercise, your children will come along. If you love yourself and nurture yourself and make time for friends and spirit and nature and family togetherness, that is what your children will take in and make a part of themselves. It's a big responsibility, sure, but that's parenting. That's being a mother. That's also what it means to live well. I know that's what you want for your family, so that's what you need to want for *you. You* are the heart, Mamas. You are the soul. Start with yourself, and your family will follow.

CHAPTER TEN

Natural Remedies from the Botanica

People who say they sleep like a baby usually don't have one.

—Leo J. Burke

I remember a particularly rough flu season in New York City. I was nannying for a high-powered, corporate-world couple, and when I arrived at their apartment that morning, their little toddler, Eva, was screaming. The mama was in a complete tizzy.

"She's been like this for two days!" she wailed. "The doctor says she just has a virus and it's not serious, but she won't stop crying and I have to get to a meeting right now!"

I looked at the panicked mama and the screaming baby and I wanted to get to the bottom of this, but there was no way that was going to happen with all that stress and noise and anxiety in the room. "Go!" I urged. "Don't worry, she'll be all right. I know just what to do."

Relieved, the mama flew out the door to her meeting and I turned and surveyed the cranky toddler, who continued to scream, although not as loudly. I smiled at her. "Are you feeling sick, baby girl? Let's fix you right up." She snuffled a little, and I wiped her runny nose. Then I took her temperature. It was slightly elevated, but nothing to warrant an emergency room visit.

With the baby on my hip, I went to the medicine cabinet to fetch the grapefruit seed extract I'd purchased the month before, knowing what a good bath additive it can be for fever. Tata always said grapefruit was "nature's antibiotic." I ran a lukewarm bath and put some of the extract in the water. In went the distraught baby, and in a few minutes, distracted by these new goings-on, she calmed down. I played with her and she splashed and even smiled a little, between fussing noises. She obviously wasn't feeling her best, but a calm, quiet atmosphere and a soothing bath were already working their magic.

When I took her out of the tub, her skin had cooled considerably. I put her down for a nap and she fell right to sleep. When she woke up, I took her temperature again. It was normal.

As it was a sunny, crisp, cool day, I knew that a little fresh air would do her a world of good. I bundled her up, tucked her into the stroller, and out we went. Sure enough, she perked up and was happy as we strolled through Central Park, singing songs from one of her favorite television programs. I looked up at the bright blue sky, smiled, and whispered, "*Gracias*, Tata!" Once again, her wisdom had guided me.

You've already listened to my lectures about what your family eats, and your diet alone can make a huge impact on your health and the strength of your immune system. When you eat well and live a healthy lifestyle, you lower your risk of illness. However, sometimes you and your children will get sick. We don't live in isolation, and we are all bound to catch the occasional virus or bacterial infection, or get a rash, or an allergy, or whatever. This is part of life. Minor illnesses shouldn't occur all the time, but they are likely to occur every now and then, even in the healthiest people.

When it comes to minor illnesses, the Organic Nanny way is to try natural remedies for symptom relief first, rather than rushing to crack open a bottle of over-the-counter medicine or begging the pediatrician for yet another dose of antibiotics (which, incidentally, do nothing against viruses, which include the common cold). Please note, I am not a doctor, and of course you should always seek professional medical care

When to Call the Doctor

If your child has a fever over 100 degrees, a serious injury, is bleeding, or is acting different than usual for no apparent reason (such as being unresponsive or hyperactive), or if you suspect your child ingested something poisonous or hit his head, or even if you just know something is wrong and you're not sure what, then please do not try to treat the problem yourself. Go to your doctor or emergency room! If you just have a feeling that it's something serious, your child's health is never worth gambling that it's probably not.

That being said, I must say that I do prefer holistic medical practitioners over conventional doctors most of the time. In my experience, holistic practitioners are more likely to look at the whole picture of a child's life, rather than just patching up the most uncomfortable or obvious of the symptoms. Holistic doctors went to medical school just like conventional doctors, but they also received training in natural methods of care. Conventional doctors are more likely (there are exceptions) to prescribe medicine without asking about lifestyle, diet, sleep patterns, or family troubles, and they also tend to give in when parents demand medicine such as antibiotics, even when those medicines aren't necessary for the child's problem.

Certainly, sometimes medicine is necessary, even lifesaving. Antibiotics are necessary for certain kinds of bacterial infections, for example. Ibuprofen or acetaminophen may be necessary to bring down a high fever. Antihistamines or even steroids might be crucial for stopping an allergic reaction.

However, many medicines are overprescribed. To stick with the antibiotics example, antibiotics can wreak havoc on a child's intestinal flora and can even lead to antibiotic resistance later on, when an antibiotic might genuinely be necessary for a serious infection. Often, a child can do fine without a harsh cough syrup or decongestant, medications that tend to have unpleasant side effects. I always opt for more conservative treatments—let the body heal itself when it can. Bodies are extremely skilled at self-healing. Simple viruses usually resolve themselves on their own with sufficient rest, fluid, and gentle whole food.

I would never expect you to play doctor, so when you are in doubt, I will say it again: Call your pediatrician. However, also be an advocate for your child's health. Ask if a medicine your doctor prescribes, such as an antibiotic, antihistamine, decongestant, or cough syrup, is actually necessary. Ask if you can try to control a mild fever with baths, rest, and fluids; a cough with a spoonful of honey; a cold with warm soup and a few days off school. If your doctor says no, your child needs medicine, then follow those instructions. But your doctor might just be relieved that you aren't demanding unnecessary medication, and she might be glad to offer you some more natural alternatives.

if you or your child is experiencing acute illness or injury, such as high fevers or extreme pain. But for minor ills, allergies, and general discomfort, I take Tata's five-step approach to healing:

1. Calm
2. Cleanse
3. Rest
4. Replenish
5. Revive

Step One: Calm

The first of Tata's five steps for healing is a big one: calm. Tata always had the most calm and peaceful demeanor. It put everyone at ease, especially children. In little Eva's case, it was obvious to me that although the baby really did have some kind of a minor virus—probably the common cold, as her pediatrician had diagnosed—the anxiety level in the household was definitely making things worse.

The best thing you can do for a sick child is to calm yourself down. Children pick up on the energy of the adults who care for them. When you radiate calm confidence, your child will calm down, too. If you aren't panicking, maybe she'll stop panicking. Be her calm comforter and her stress level will go down. That will give her immune system a better chance to take care of the problem. Our bodies are wise healers, if we will only get out of the way.

Organic Voices

To insure good health: eat lightly, breathe deeply, live moderately, cultivate cheerfulness, and maintain an interest in life.

—*William London*

I understand you are worried. Or hurried. But take a deep breath, Mamas. Calm yourself, and then listen to your child. You'll be much more likely to hear her, pick up on the subtle signs of an imbalance, and know what to do if you have a calm mind, and I can guarantee it will make your child feel a little bit better. Whether we are sick or not, stress makes us all feel worse.

Step Two: Cleanse

No matter what the problem, Tata always recommended some type of cleansing—water, inside and out, with or without the help of natural herbs, is an excellent way to help set the body right again.

Cleansing helps cool the skin and flush toxins from the system. With children, this must be a gentle, natural process, and my favorite way to do this with children is to "prescribe" a bath.

Tata used to give people bath salts or infusions from herbs, like big tea bags for the bathtub. I still do this today. Soaking in a warm bath that is properly infused with herbs and salts gently draws toxins out through the skin, relaxes the muscles, and calms the mind. This is especially important if your child is on antibiotics. A bath may help draw excess medicine out of the skin. If you are still working to phase out conventional food, this can also help to cleanse the body of antibiotics and other toxins you may have ingested from factory-farmed animals and dairy products.

A bath can also help bring down a fever, invigorate a child who has the blues, or calm an anxious or hyperactive child. I've seen many stresses as well as minor illnesses gently coaxed away through the magical ritual of the bath.

Better Baths

Water alone is a lovely cleanser, but there are ways Tata taught me to increase the healing and cleansing power of the bath. One is to use essential oils in bathwater, for an aromatherapy effect. Certain aromas can have very specific effects on the body and the emotions. While essential oils should be diluted for use with children, and kept out of eyes, nose, and mouth, they can be incredibly soothing and therapeutic. Just two or three drops in a child's warm bathwater should do the trick. Here are some essential oils I like to use for specific issues (look for organic varieties in your natural foods store or health store):

- *Fever, minor cuts, fungal infections (e.g., athlete's foot):* any citrus (grapefruit, lemon, orange)

La Botanica

La botanica was my Tata's home away from home. In Cuban slang, a *botanica* is a natural pharmacy for anything that ails you—it's full of herbs, poultices, tonics, and other traditional folk remedies, along with spiritual inspiration in the form of candles, icons, and other little things relevant and inspiring to the Latino community. You might also find some Asian remedies at *la botanica*—there is actually a fairly large Chinese population in Cuba.

You may not have a botanica in your neighborhood, but you can begin to collect your own nontoxic natural remedies right in your own medicine cabinet. Turn first to these, rather than all those medicines—the cold remedies, cough syrups, pain relievers, all those things that have side effects that can be worse than the actual problem they are supposedly relieving.

- *Skin irritation (e.g., rashes and insect bites):* lavender, chamomile, tea tree
- *Nausea/upset stomach:* peppermint, fennel, chamomile
- *Anxiety, hyperactivity:* chamomile, jasmine, mandarin, lavender
- *Sadness:* geranium, rose, peppermint, ylang-ylang

Another way to make a bath a more productively cleansing experience is with a bath tea bag. Cut a big square of cheesecloth (about one foot along each side) and fill it with herbs. Drop it in the bathtub as the water is running, and the herbs will infuse the bathwater. When the bath is over, just throw your "tea bag" away. Here are some herbs I like to include in a general cleansing bath for children. You should be able to find them at your local natural food stores, in the bulk herb section (often located next to the bulk tea):

- Orange leaves (*hojas de naranja*)
- Mint leaves (*hojas de menta*)
- Linden leaves (*tilo*)

- Dandelion root
- Echinacea
- Lavender flowers

Finally, a cup of Epsom salts in the bath will make the water feel silky-soft, making the bath more relaxing and pleasurable for kids (or for you!). It may also help calm and soothe anxious children, and some parents say it is of particular benefit to their autistic children. Also, a teaspoon of olive oil and a half cup of oat flour (put dry oatmeal in your blender to turn it into flour) stirred into bathwater will help soothe dry, itchy skin.

Pooping Is Vital!

I will never forget little Lawrence. The toddler son of a Manhattan stockbroker and an older mother who doted on and constantly worried about him, Lawrence suffered from constipation. His mother told me that he would scream with pain, and for some mysterious reason, the only time he would have a bowel movement was when I was there on the weekends. Lawrence had a different nanny during the week, and he was with his parents in the evenings.

What was I doing differently? His mother couldn't understand it. The doctor had given them a special prescription laxative powder, at the price of $180, but it didn't seem to be working very well and she worried about the harsh effects. She was desperate to find an answer and to soothe her baby's pain. She worried that he might have some kind of gastrointestinal disease.

I had my suspicions, but I didn't want to point any fingers, so I suggested we make a chart to find out what everybody was feeding him. Since Lawrence had several different caregivers, I told his mother we needed to see if we could find any patterns.

Sure enough, the nanny who took care of Lawrence during the week was giving him fast-food for lunch. I also discovered, through listening, that the poor little guy's environment was extremely stressful. He seemed to be picking up on the anxiety of his parents.

What was I doing differently? When I arrived each Saturday morning, I began by giving Lawrence a quiet bath. When I picked him up, I could just feel how overwhelmed this little guy was. He was tense and anxious, but he soon began to calm down in the warm bath.

After the bath, I would make Lawrence a special juice drink, just for him. I included a little bit of prune juice, which softens the bowels, along with some cherry juice and a squeeze of lemon. He would drink this juice, and within an hour, he would have a nice healthy poop. "Look!" I said to his mother one Saturday afternoon. "I just saved you $180."

For the rest of the day, Lawrence drank water and ate healthy plant foods (no French fries!). He was calm and happy and he never screamed. I wasn't working any miracles—I was just helping this poor little boy's body along a bit. When I explained all this to his mother, she immediately told the other nanny to adopt this new routine. In just a few days, Lawrence became a calmer, quieter, happy child—and all his constipation issues dissolved.

Listen to me, Mamas: pooping is vital! It is your body's internal cleansing mechanism. A good, healthy daily poop will help your child feel better, and it all starts with a clean diet of fiber-rich plant foods, plenty of water, and no junk food! The plant food part alone can make a huge difference in regularity. Add calm and cleansing, and you'll have things running relatively smoothly in no time.

When things still get a little backed up, as they sometimes do, especially during stressful times, try this natural remedy, the one I used with Lawrence and my go-to remedy whenever a child complains of a tummy ache and I know he hasn't pooped in a while:

Tata's Smooth Move Juice Remedy

3 ounces organic apple juice
3 ounces purified water
3 ounces organic prune juice
3 tablespoons organic black cherry juice
1 tablespoon organic flaxseed oil

Mix all the ingredients and serve cold.

Castor Oil Massage

Tata always used another remedy on my brother and me when we were little and had a stomachache: She would rub castor oil on our tummy before bed, paying particular attention to the area over the liver. It always worked—and it was so much nicer than having to swallow the stuff! In the morning, the body will release what it is holding on to.

And don't forget your teeth. Keeping teeth clean is so important for overall health, but although we clean our teeth, we may forget to clean our toothbrushes! Replace toothbrushes about every three months to minimize the accumulation of bacteria.

Drink Up

Finally, let's not forget the most important key to basic internal cleansing: water! Hydration is crucial. Many children don't get enough fluids in their diet, and when a child is sick, he needs extra hydration to help his body flush out viruses and bacteria.

Many children also learn to enjoy gentle, weak herbal tea. The ritual of a warm cup of tea can be comforting and calming, as well as hydrating. Try these teas for what ails your child:

- *For calming:* chamomile (unless your child is allergic to ragweed), spearmint, cinnamon, hibiscus
- *For upset tummies:* ginger, peppermint, fennel
- *For sore throats:* lemon or orange tea with a spoonful of raw honey (do not give honey to children under one year old)
- *For stuffy noses:* echinacea (don't use long term, just while your child has a cold), peppermint, orange. (And remember, dairy products increase congestion, so especially when your child has a head cold, skip the dairy products!)

Clear soups are also excellent for hydration.

Always offer children plenty of fresh water. Pure, clean water is the best way to hydrate, and is so important for healing. When a child has a cold or a fever, or you just want to help head off that virus going around the school, be sure he is drinking extra water. Drink it cool, or warm with a squeeze of lemon and a spoonful of honey, especially to ease coughing. Water can help bring down a fever, ease sticky congestion, soothe a cough, and help the body work better. It helps flush toxins through the digestive system and can combat dehydration your child might experience due to fever or diarrhea. Encourage your children to sip water all day, and always serve water with meals. Keep a pitcher in the refrigerator for easy do-it-yourself hydration. A few lemon, lime, or orange slices in the pitcher can add a bit of flavor.

Step Three: Rest

Sleep is an amazing healer, and it is an important step in the healing process. After your ill child is cleansed and hydrated inside and out, let her take a nap. If she can't sleep, just urge her to lie still and close her eyes. Most of us can use more sleep, and children who don't feel well need it most of all, especially if they are feeling anxious or have worn themselves out with fussing. The body heals best during sleep.

In fact, children who get regular sleep may be in better shape to fight off illness in the first place, but many children don't get enough. Did you know that lack of sleep has been linked to cause the following in children:

- Attention problems
- Memory problems
- Anxiety
- Obesity

There is nothing wrong with taking a nap in the middle of the day, if you need it (and that includes you, Mamas!). But for some children, as well as many adults, sleep is elusive. Many children have bedtime issues.

Organic Nanny Notes

Your child may need more sleep than you think, and most kids don't get enough. According to the National Sleep Foundation, this is how much sleep children generally require each night for good health and best mental functioning (children under a lot of stress may need more, and a few may do fine on a little less):

- Newborns up to 2 months old: 12 to 18 hours
- Infants 3 to 11 months old: 14 to 15 hours
- Toddlers 1 to 3 years old: 12 to 14 hours
- Preschoolers 3 to 5 years old: 11 to 13 hours
- Children 5 to 10 years old: 10 to 11 hours
- Teens 10 to 17 years old: 8 1/2 to 9 1/4 hours
- Adults 18 years and older: 7 to 9 hours

When your child has trouble getting to sleep, try these Organic Nanny Sleepytime Strategies:

- Be sure your child gets some exercise earlier in the day, but not too close to bedtime. After dinner, keep the household calm. When dinner has been cleaned up, it's time to start getting ready for bedtime.
- Make bedtime a ritual. Children crave rituals. When you do about the same thing every night in the same order at the same time, your child will know what to expect, and the very process will be calming and more likely to induce sleep. Change is exciting. Ritual is calming.
- A warm bath is a great way to begin. Don't rush, stay calm, and encourage quieter play. Try playing relaxing music during bathtime, to help set a calmer mood.
- Turn off the television at least one hour before bedtime. Let this time be family time, with actual conversation and hugs and eye contact. But no arguing!

- Try massage, which induces a relaxation response. Sing softly to your child or play gentle music while rubbing her shoulders, hands, and feet. Use gentle pressure on muscles, but ask your child to tell you if she wants a lighter or deeper massage.
- Put together an Organic Nanny Sleepytime Tray for each child. I use this with many of my clients, and it works like a charm. Find a wooden tray, or better yet, let your child help you hunt for one in antique stores, thrift stores, or craft stores. You can paint it with your child's name, and she can help decorate it. This special tray is only for use during the bedtime ritual. Every night, prepare the Sleepytime Tray (or call it something else that appeals to your child). Include:
  - A snack. Good bedtime snacks might include a cut-up apple or pear; a glass of water or nondairy milk; and a small, naturally sweetened organic cookie, or a few crackers with peanut butter. Keep it sugar and caffeine free and don't forget that your child should brush her teeth afterwards!
  - A storybook.
  - A toy to snuggle with.
  - A CD of gentle background music.
  - Anything else your child needs before sleep or during the night.

You can vary what is on the tray, but use the tray every night for a dependable and calming part of the bedtime ritual.

- Read to your child. A bedtime story is an age-old ritual that really works to put kids in a sleepy frame of mind. This is a great chance for papas to step in, as many of them make excellent storytellers. Just remind the teller to keep things relatively low-key. A rousing adventure story can be great fun for the feel-good evenings, or for daytime stories, but not on those nights when a good night's sleep is essential. For sick children in particular, soothing stories are best.
- Spray the underside of your child's pillow with lavender spray, which is calming and encourages sleep. Or, if this seems too strong, just spritz a corner of the room.

Apple Kudzu Drink

Apple kudzu makes an excellent bedtime drink for the Sleepytime Tray. My children love apple kudzu, which we drink instead of hot cocoa. Kudzu is the dried, flaked root of the kudzu plant, and in folk medicine it is known for its ability to relieve intestinal cramps. It also seems to calm the nervous system, so it's especially good for calming hyperactive or overstimulated children. It's also thought to fight fevers. If I suspect one of my children is coming down with something, the first thing I do is break out the kudzu!

Put 1 cup of apple juice in a small saucepan and gently heat it to a low boil. As the apple juice is heating, combine 1 tablespoon of flaked kudzu with about 1/4 cup of water. When the apple juice boils, pour in the kudzu mixture and stir until the kudzu is dissolved into the apple juice. Pour into two to four small cups and let the apple kudzu cool to a safe temperature for sipping.

You can find kudzu in your natural foods store, or order it online.

- Teach your child deep breathing, an instant calmer. Together, inhale slowly to the count of five, then exhale slowly to the count of five. (If five counts are too long, try three.) Do this ten times before bed every night. Deep breathing actually signals the nervous system to relax.
- Have a final good-night saying. Whether it's "Love you always!" or "Nighty-night" or "Sweet dreams for my sweet baby!" always say the same thing just before you leave the room. It should be something calm and sweet and full of love (no talk of biting bedbugs, please!). It will become a signal to your child that this will be your final contact before morning, and that feels comforting.
- Finally, after your child is asleep, use these tips on yourself! You're probably not getting enough sleep, either. You can even have your own grown-up version of a Sleepytime Tray, with herbal tea, a good book, and a lavender eye pillow. You might be tempted to add a

glass of wine, but this can actually disrupt sleep rhythms, so it's not a good bedtime drink if you are having sleep issues. Turn off the TV and calm your mind. Read a book, or meditate. Take some long, slow, deep breaths, and turn in early.

Your Child's Bed vs. Your Bed

I've always been a fan of and practitioner of the principles of attachment parenting, a system of raising children that encourages physical contact and intuition. One of the original principles of attachment parenting is co-sleeping. That means that sleeping with your baby is not just okay but encouraged. It makes middle-of-the-night nursing easier, and it helps maintain that close physical bond between parent and child.

At some point as your child gets older, however, you may decide that it is time for him to transition to his own bed. When this happens (and whether your child sleeps with you at all) is up to you and should be based on your own feelings and intuition, not on what someone else tells you that you should be doing. When you feel you and your child are ready, however, you might make a cute "I Slept in My Own Bed!" chart, to help reward your child for his successes.

Every night your child stays in his own bed all night long, he gets a gold star on the chart. After ten, twenty, or thirty nights with stars, he gets a special prize—a new toy, perhaps, or a special day with you doing something he loves. This is a fun way to reward good behavior, rather than punishing your child when he gets anxious and comes into your room.

Punishing causes more anxiety, making your child feel less confident about staying in his own room, and I simply do not advocate it. I believe it makes sleep issues worse, not better. When staying put becomes rewarding, a sign to your child that he is getting older and more capable of taking care of some of his own needs, he may feel more motivated to do it.

Still, I urge you not to feel pressure to conform to someone else's idea of where your child should be sleeping. Co-sleeping is a perfectly lovely way to bond, but it's not for everyone. Only you know when it's right, and only you know when it's time to move on to the next stage. Listen to your heart on this one, Mamas.

Once you begin making the transition, please know that it is normal for toddlers to periodically run out of their room and into yours at night. Most parents regard this as a normal developmental stage, though these night visits can be exhausting for you.

To give your child extra nighttime security without disrupting your sleep, put a futon, mattress, or sleeping bag at the foot of your bed, then explain to your child that she may come into your room at night only if she sleeps in her special bed, and as long as she can tiptoe as quiet as a mouse so she doesn't wake you up. Explain that mommies (and daddies) need their sleep; that a good sleep is very, very important; and that without a good sleep, sometimes parents can become cranky in the morning. Coming into your room without waking you is good practice for your child, and will help her feel even more confident in her ability to control her own nighttime behavior. Eventually, that confidence will keep her in her big-girl bed.

Other ways to entice your child to stay in his own room and bed:

- Leave a glass of water at his bedside in case he wakes up thirsty.
- Put on a continuous-play tape recording of you singing a medley of lullabies.
- Make his bed so attractive that he wants to stay in it, by letting him pick out a special comforter, sheets, or sleeping bag, and allowing him to bring favorite toys under the covers.
- Don't be stuck in the "kids shouldn't do that" mentality when you don't really have a good reason. If he really wants to bring a flashlight into his bed and it makes him feel safer, then why not? If he wants to sleep with his head at the foot of the bed, then let him have that power over his own environment. Routine is important, but so is giving your child freedom to be himself. (The only exception is if he wants to do something you know will keep him from getting a good night's sleep, such as leave every light on, play music loudly, or watch television. Only you can judge what will and will not be conducive to sleep for each individual child, but studies do show that lights, noise, and flickering screens compromise sleep quality.)

The attachment-parenting way of going to sleep—a close physical bond with you—is particularly helpful if you have an active child who has trouble settling down. Besides, what baby or toddler would choose to be alone in a dark room instead of snuggled at his mother's breast? Don't worry that letting your child sleep with you, or fall asleep on you before you put him in his crib, will cause him any harm or "spoil" him. On the contrary, it will make him feel safer and more confident (despite what your mother or neighbor or best friend might tell you).

Step Four: Replenish

A calm, clean, well-rested child will heal quickly, but you can do even more to help combat minor illness by giving the body more of what it needs: nutrition and natural remedies. Most minor illnesses can be managed at home with gentle healthy foods and natural remedies. Here's what Tata taught me:

For the Common Cold

One of the most common childhood ailments is the common cold—I don't know any child who gets through childhood without catching the occasional cold virus. However, you don't have to treat a cold with over-the-counter cough syrups, decongestants, and antihistamines. There are better ways to relieve the symptoms of a child's cold.

For stuffy noses, fill a bowl with steaming water. Add four drops of tea tree oil and four drops of eucalyptus essential oil. Stay with your child and have her lean over the bowl, but not so close that she feels uncomfortable. Drape a towel over her head and the bowl. Sit with and rub her back for ten minutes. The steam will help loosen congestion.

For coughs, this homemade cough syrup is easy to make and helps even the most stubborn little coughs. It also helps clear out congestion. This recipe is a gentle and effective alternative to overpriced commercial cough syrups, and it contains no artificial ingredients. (Note: This recipe uses honey. Honey is not technically vegan, but because it has natural cough suppressant properties, I prefer it as a medicine to pharmaceutical cough syrups, which contain drugs and often alcohol. If you can buy honey from a small-scale local beekeeper, that is ideal. If you are opposed to honey, use maple syrup instead. The sweet syrup itself can help relieve coughs, even if it doesn't have all the properties of honey.)

Organic Nanny Cough Syrup
(for children over 1 year old)

2 cups purified water
1 tablespoon powdered slippery elm (find it in natural health food
    stores or through www.mountainroseherbs.com)
1/2 teaspoon ground ginger
1/4 cup raw honey
Juice from 1 organic lemon

Combine the water, slippery elm, and ginger in a saucepan. Heat on low heat until the liquid comes to a boil. Continue to boil until the liquid is reduced by half. Remove from the heat and stir in the honey and lemon juice. Store in a clean glass bottle in the refrigerator. Give your child 2 tablespoons, up to four times per day.

For Skin Irritation and Dryness

Just as the body needs liquid, so does the skin. A bath is great for hydrating skin, but you can also use natural emollients on dry or irritated skin to soothe it and make it feel good. Sometimes when children get sick, they get very dry skin and chapped lips. One of my favorite Cuban remedies is cacao butter. You can use it on every part of your skin, including chapped lips. It smells and tastes like chocolate because it is made from chocolate. You can buy raw cacao butter at Whole Foods and other natural foods stores, or find it online at www.sunfood.com. It can be pricey, but a little goes a long way and a jar will last you for many months or even years if you use it sparingly.

For a rash or irritated skin, try fresh aloe vera gel. It can heal insect bites, patches of dry skin, and sunburns. The best way to use it is straight from the plant. Keep an aloe plant or two in your home and tend it well. To use it, tear off the tip of a leaf and rub the gel from inside the leaf onto the affected part of the skin. It's gentle, pure, and nontoxic when used externally, so it's even fine for little faces.

You can also treat skin from the inside. I love almond milk for dry skin, acne, and chapped lips. Almond milk contains vitamins A and E, which contribute to softer skin. It's also great for teenagers because it combats breakouts with its high concentration of essential fatty acids, which have a beautifying effect on the complexion. You can use almond milk in place of dairy milk in just about any situation. Make the switch and your whole family will enjoy smoother, softer skin and less acne after just one week. Try it!

Finally, Tata had a secret recipe for skin cream that she always kept in the house for us to use. I swear by it. It includes calendula (marigold), an herb that has remarkable skin-healing properties. Tata mixed it by hand according to "feel" and never measured, but this is my closest approximation to what she did. This cream is hypoallergenic and makes an excellent salve for dry skin, rashes, and eczema. You should be able to find all these ingredients from your natural foods store.

Tata's Cuban Calendula Skin Cream _____

2 tablespoons calendula oil
2 tablespoons water
2 tablespoons aloe vera gel
2 tablespoons virgin coconut oil
10 drops French lavender oil
4 tablespoons sweet almond oil

Mix all the ingredients together and store in a glass jar. Use as needed.

If you don't want to make your own calendula cream, California Baby makes a similar product. You can find it online at www.californiababy

.com. Or, try the company's Everyday French Lavender lotion. California Baby was created by Mama Jessica in her kitchen. Its products contain no gluten, soy, oat, dairy, or nuts (except for coconut, which is really a seed). Everything is made with cold-pressed vegan oils and pure essential-oil blends. All the oils are organic and the products are never animal tested. This company's products are the closest thing I've found to what Tata made herself—and you can even purchase them at Target!

Step Five: Revitalize!

The final step in my Organic Nanny cure is to let Mother Nature have direct access to your child. There is no better way to revitalize a tired, cranky, sick, or uncomfortable child than with fresh air and sunlight.

After the calm, the cleanse, the rest, and the replenish, dress your child appropriately for the weather and take a short, relaxing stroll outside, or just sit outside in the sun for a few minutes. Wrap the child in a blanket or not. Sometimes sick children will feel especially privileged if you set up a comfy spot just for them out on the porch or deck, and they are allowed to sit out there in their pajamas and slippers. Special! Even fifteen minutes of fresh air and sunshine with deep healing breaths can make your child feel like she's on the mend.

Don't Forget L.O.V.E.

So much of this book is about food that I didn't spend time talking about it in this chapter. You already know that eating L.O.V.E. foods—local, organic, vegan or vegetarian, and environmentally friendly—will help bring your body back into balance. A poor diet weakens the body, making it more susceptible to disease. A good diet full of vibrant, vitamin-rich plant foods strengthens the body and the immune system to best fight off any illnesses that come your children's way. So this is just a gentle reminder— eat well, Mamas, and feed your children well, too, to keep them as healthy as they can be. You may find they get sick much less often on a whole plant foods diet.

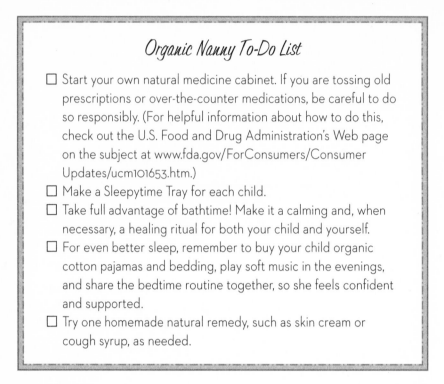

Organic Nanny To-Do List

☐ Start your own natural medicine cabinet. If you are tossing old prescriptions or over-the-counter medications, be careful to do so responsibly. (For helpful information about how to do this, check out the U.S. Food and Drug Administration's Web page on the subject at www.fda.gov/ForConsumers/Consumer Updates/ucm101653.htm.)

☐ Make a Sleepytime Tray for each child.

☐ Take full advantage of bathtime! Make it a calming and, when necessary, a healing ritual for both your child and yourself.

☐ For even better sleep, remember to buy your child organic cotton pajamas and bedding, play soft music in the evenings, and share the bedtime routine together, so she feels confident and supported.

☐ Try one homemade natural remedy, such as skin cream or cough syrup, as needed.

Nobody wants a sick baby, toddler, grade-schooler—or, heaven forbid, a sick teenager! (I find they tend to complain the loudest about their discomfort.) We all worry about sniffles, coughs, rashes, and general crankiness, but see your doctor when necessary, and follow these five steps. I guarantee you'll be doing everything you can to speed your child's healing.

CHAPTER ELEVEN

An Attitude of Gratitude

Be thankful for what you have; you'll end up having more.
If you concentrate on what you don't have,
you will never, ever have enough.

—Oprah Winfrey

One very balmy summer in New York, I was hired to nanny for a stunning, high-profile fashion model from Spain who asked me to call her "Señora." Señora was the most strikingly gorgeous woman I'd ever seen. Her skin was absolutely amazing. She spoke with a true Castilian accent, substituting her *s* letters with the *th* sound; for example, *cinco* and *siesta* were "thinco" and "thiethta," as she pronounced them in her wonderfully buttery voice. She exuded European flair.

Señora was a single mom to a beautiful eight-year-old daughter named Sierra. Señora was often away because she worked mostly in Europe and Japan, but her home base was a fabulous loft in downtown Manhattan.

Even as a child, Señora loved animals more than she loved most people, and preferred not to eat meat. She used to swap her chicken and beef for her brother's vegetables. You might think from looking at her as an adult that she would be fastidious about her household, but because Señora was a huge animal lover, the house was full of pets.

That meant I was not just Sierra's nanny—I also became caretaker to a menagerie, which included Gato, a big, fat, cranky white cat; two bunnies named Bunny A and Bunny B; Rollie, the distinguished dachshund; and a Vietnamese pot-bellied piglet named Gus. Even when Sierra napped, it was impossible to be lonely in that household.

All the animals were sweet (except for Gato, who would purr like a motorboat and then turn on me without warning, claws poised like little daggers), but Gus in particular was an angel in a piglet's body. Señora bought him at an upstate farmers' market when he was two months old. He snorted with gusto and always wanted to cuddle, which was fine as at this point he only weighed about 20 pounds (later in his life, he'd come close to 150). He acted like a puppy, slept in a crate, and loved to have his belly scratched. Sierra would dress him up in her old toddler clothes and Gus would just snort with glee and roll over onto his back. He'd lie down with me if I took a nap and would jump up and run to the door if he heard the bell—such a "guard pig" he was! I was amazed by his loyalty and intelligence, and had as much fun with him as I did with Sierra.

During our summer together, Sierra came to a very grown-up conclusion on her own: She said she wanted to become a vegetarian because she couldn't imagine eating her best friend, Gus. Señora had not been feeding Sierra a vegetarian diet because she didn't want to impose her beliefs on her daughter, but was proud of her child's decision, and of course I was, too. Children often decide on their own to go the way of their parents, especially when they aren't forced to comply to something they don't like or understand. The daily menus were altered and meat was banished from the home completely.

Years later, Sierra became an animal rights and environmental activist in New York City. When I heard that, I couldn't help but smile because I knew in my heart that Gus had a whole lot to do with that.

Gratitude 101

You may have taught your children to say, "Thank you," when someone does something for them, and they may repeat the words out of habit and conditioning, but how well do your children really understand gratitude? Many of the children I've met and cared for take their easy life circumstances for granted, and why shouldn't they? They don't know what it means to be poor or neglected or to have to do without. Those children are lucky . . . but are they grateful?

And, why do I bring up this story about Señora and Sierra and their menagerie now, in a chapter about gratitude?

I believe that animals are some of our greatest teachers, and they provide a wonderful opportunity to teach children about gratitude. Just as they are attracted to the stuffed toy ones, something draws children to a live puppy or a kitten or a bird or a small animal. Our pets love us no matter how we look or act or what our social standing is in life. And children can easily sense this unconditional love. I believe that whether you are a vegetarian or not, you can use their relationship with animals as a way to help them understand what it means to give without expectation or condition, and by extension, to appreciate unconditional giving from others. Beginning with animals is such a sweet way to draw children into an attitude of gratitude. Children's natural affinity for animals is the starting point for teaching reverence for all life, from annoying siblings to friends to all people and animals on the planet—and for the planet itself.

Children may take for granted that their parents will love them and care for them. Many of the children I've nannied are incredibly privileged, and grow up believing they deserve to get whatever they want. However, when someone who doesn't have to loves them and shows them affection—especially when they are chosen by an animal—they are filled with wonderment. It only takes one little extra step to bring your child's attention to this, and to ask her what we might do in return to give back to animals. Sharing and giving help to an animal feels a lot easier and more effortless than sharing or giving unconditionally to a sibling or another child, or to a cause a child might not understand.

What are some ways to help your children practice "giving back" to animals?

- Take your children to visit pets at an animal shelter. Older children might even want to volunteer, walking dogs and playing with cats.

Surf the Web for Animal Rights

These organizations work tirelessly to defend the right of animals to live lives of dignity, free from suffering. Find out more about them via their informative Web sites:

- People for the Ethical Treatment of Animals (PETA): www.peta.org
- Compassion over Killing (COK): www.cok.net
- Farm Sanctuary: www.farmsanctuary.org
- The Humane Society of the United States (HSUS): www.humansociety.org
- American Society for the Prevention of Cruelty to Animals (ASPCA): www.aspca.org

- Consider adopting a pet. If you don't have a pet and you think your family is ready for the responsibility, consider adopting a pet that has lost its home. Growing up with pets is an excellent way for children to learn compassion and responsibility (although a pet's care should always ultimately be the adult's responsibility, never the children's, just for the sake of the animal).
- Encourage your children to donate their allowance or lemonade stand proceeds to the local animal shelter or another animal organization. One little boy I know recently had a birthday party, and requested on the invitation that he receive no presents, only that the guests donate to the local animal shelter. I was so proud of him!
- Eat more plant foods and fewer (or no) animal foods!

Thanks, Mother Nature!

Another easy way to help your children begin to understand gratitude is to spend more time outdoors together. Children spend so much time now in front of the computer, the television, or the video game console that they forget how beautiful and giving the natural world can be. As denizens of Earth, we are all given the gift of sun and wind and blue sky and water and green trees and plants and beautiful wild animals everywhere, from birds and squirrels to deer and fox, snakes and bugs and fish and more, depending on where you live. Exposure to the natural world opens up a child's mind in a way no video game or text messaging conversation ever could.

Encourage children to appreciate and give back to nature by picking up litter when they see it (and of course, never littering themselves!), donating time or money to local environmental organizations, and learning as much as they can about nature. Many young environmental scientists were created out of a passion for learning about the natural world.

Organic Voices

Research has shown that a simple act of kindness directed towards another improves the functioning of the immune system and stimulates the production of serotonin in both the recipient of kindness and the person extending kindness. Even more amazing is that persons observing the act of kindness have similar beneficial results. Imagine this! Kindness extended, received, or observed beneficially impacts the physical health and feeling of everyone involved.

—Dr. Wayne Dyer

A Day of Service

Learning to serve others is such a crucial skill for children, who are often so used to being served. Many children reach adulthood without ever purposefully going out of their own way to help someone else. You can instill a sense of gratitude through service in your children so easily, and I hope you will do this. It builds character, integrity, compassion, and an appreciation for all life: human, animal, even plant life, if service is geared toward environmental preservation.

To integrate the concept of service in the household, I suggest instituting a monthly or even weekly Day of Service. On that day, you and your children set out to help someone who needs it. Make a plan and then make it happen.

A Day of Service can be of huge benefit to a child. When a child is bored and demands to be entertained, perhaps that is a red flag that she is more than ready to learn that others are much less fortunate than she is, and that she can do something about it to help.

How you plan your Day of Service depends on how much time you have, but however you do it, make it a priority. Your child could change the world! Here are some ideas for ways to integrate service into your family:

Visit a nursing home.

In Cuban culture, we live in multigenerational households and we all care for our aging relatives. This is common in Asian cultures, too. Here, however, so many older people live isolated and alone, discarded from a society that finds their increasing needs inconvenient.

So many of them would delight in a visit from a child. Children who don't know anyone who is older may learn to fear the very old, and what a shame that is. Children who meet and interact with older folks regularly learn to love and appreciate them, and to learn from their wisdom (which is vast). Especially if your child doesn't have an opportunity to interact regularly with his own grandparents or great-grandparents, you could make senior center visits a regular activity you and your child do together.

Organic Voices

The way you get meaning into your life is to devote yourself to loving others, devote yourself to your community around you, and devote yourself to creating something that gives you purpose and meaning.

—*Mitch Albom*

(Screen the senior center first by visiting once by yourself. Some environments may be too startling for children, which is even sadder for those who have to live in them.)

Volunteer at a soup kitchen.

Many communities have soup kitchens or other resources to feed people who don't have enough to eat. Many of these also allow families to volunteer. I know a family who spends every Thanksgiving feeding the hungry at a local soup kitchen. Since the children in the family were old enough to walk, they would come along to help, even just to pass out dinner rolls. What a wonderful idea! (And no cooking for the mama!) Children who have plenty to eat, even the luxury to buy organic produce and choose to be vegan, can learn an important lesson about the world when they see people who simply can't afford to have dinner at all. It opens their minds and they come to an attitude of gratitude all on their own.

Do trail maintenance.

Many local parks and recreation areas need regular maintenance of trails and other natural areas, and are in dire need of community volunteers to help. Take your family along and help clear and maintain these valuable natural areas. It's fun, it's a day outside in the fresh air, and you are helping preserve the natural world. Contact your local park service to find out about volunteer opportunities.

Help animal shelters.

Many local animal shelters and humane societies need help because they are underfunded and understaffed. Helping is fun and easy, too. Many need people to walk the dogs, pet and socialize the cats, and clean cages. Although young children shouldn't be cleaning any cages, they can certainly come along and interact with the animals, if the shelter allows. Talk to your local shelter about what they need and you and your child could help. Even if that just means donating a box of supplies, you and your child can choose them together and deliver them to the shelter.

Donate for the holidays.

During the holiday season, many parents don't have the resources to buy gifts for their children, or even warm coats, boots, and mittens. Many communities have drives, such as Toys for Tots, which collect new toys and other gifts for children in need, and/or warm winter clothing. This is a great way to involve your child, who can certainly understand the importance of holiday gifts and warm mittens on a cold winter day. Let her help you choose toys for another child (a great lesson in itself for children who get a little too excited about what they will be getting), as well as boots, coats, mittens, hats, and scarves.

Take service vacations.

I'm seeing more and more service vacations geared toward families. Some of these are more appropriate when your child is older, and may travel abroad or stay right here in the United States. The Sierra Club (www.sierraclub.org) is famous for service vacations that help restore the natural environment, but other groups have service vacations that help children, provide health-care services, work with teens or seniors, or help the hungry. Just be sure to research the organization first, and get recommendations. One organization I like is Global Volunteers (www .globalvolunteers.org). This organization places volunteers with volunteer projects around the world. Their Web site has a section called Family Volunteering, with a chart showing the minimum age required for volunteers in each country or area (many allow children to come along who are as young as six or eight). Their motto is "Travel that feeds the soul."

Volunteer with your dog!

Many people have trained their dogs to become therapy dogs. Therapy dogs go with you to hospitals and nursing homes visiting sick or injured children or lonely seniors. Something about petting a dog seems to promote healing and balance in people who are in pain or feeling isolated. I've even heard true firsthand stories about people who awoke from comas or children who finally spoke after a trauma, just because they visited with a dog! Animals have such power.

If your dog is calm, sociable, and sensitive (as many dogs are), check with local hospitals or nursing homes to find out about their requirements for service animals. Many require dogs to be certified therapy dogs, but certification isn't all that difficult. Contact Therapy Dogs International

---

Gratitude Journal

A study at the University of California at Davis compared families who journaled about things they were thankful for with those who journaled about the daily things that bothered or irritated them. The families who journaled about gratitude had fewer signs of illness and reported feeling better about their lives in the present and more optimistic about their future. What a great practice! Start a gratitude journal, and encourage your child to start one, too. This could become part of your evening routine—bring out the journal before bed and jot down one thing you are both grateful for that day, whether it's a cuddly kitten, an extra-long bedtime story, a good day at school, or cookies! If you or your child already keep a diary, this is an easy thing to add to each entry.

(www.tdi-dog.org), Therapy Dogs Inc. (www.therapydogs.com), or the Delta Society (www.deltasociety.org) for more information about how to get your dog certified as a therapy dog (often, all it takes is an evaluation or a training class). Take your child along on your visits (if allowed by the facility), and you'll brighten the days of those who need it with both your dog and your child.

Even if your Day of Service happens just once a year (although I hope it will happen more often), there are so many opportunities out there for character building, and so many people and animals in need, that I hope you will adopt this family tradition. And if you can't find a volunteer opportunity that children can participate in? Maybe it's time you started one! Contact local organizations, such as food banks, battered woman shelters, or soup kitchens, to find out what they think is the greatest area of need in your community affecting children, animals, or people your child can relate to—and then see if you can fill it together!

Beyond Thanksgiving

Many families pause before Thanksgiving dinner to think about or even say out loud what they are thankful for, but why limit this practice

---

Just Say Thank You

Teaching small children to say, "Thank you," to others whenever they are given something may seem like a minor ritual required by our culture, but I believe it is more than that. Just saying the words *thank you* has an effect on children, even if they don't consciously recognize it or they say the words out of habit. I see so many children today, especially older ones, who barely grunt an acknowledgment when someone does something for them. The grateful teenager who looks an adult in the eye and says, "Thank you," with sincerity may be a rare sight in the twenty-first century, but that doesn't mean a concerted effort by concerned organic mamas can't bring it back into fashion. The best way to do this is to remind children gently, and of course, to be an excellent model of the behavior yourself. Thank you: say it, mean it, live it—and watch your life change.

---

to one day a year? Long ago, most families said grace before a meal, which in essence was a daily expression of gratitude for the good things they had. When you focus on what you don't have, you become increasingly dissatisfied—and I know that is not something you want for your child.

So focus on what you have, every day. Why not reinstitute the tradition of grace? It doesn't have to be religious, if that doesn't resonate with your family. Whenever you sit down to a meal, no matter how informal—before you ever take a bite of food—make a new habit. Say aloud, or at least think about, what you are grateful for in that moment: God's blessings, the food on your table, a warm home, people who love you, a beautiful child, an adoring pet, money to pay your bills, good friends, warm clothing, an education, the fact that you are having cupcakes for dessert. Big or small, noble or silly, find something, and acknowledge it. It can change your life—and make your children even more beautiful people than they already are.

Ideally, let the whole family participate. When your entire family sits down for dinner, pass the gratitude before you pass the mashed potatoes. Kids may balk at first, but a habit established is a powerful thing, so persevere. They may soon learn to not just say they are grateful for food and family and love and shelter, but to actually *feel* it.

Remember, a deep and sincere sense of gratitude is a gift. Someday, your children may pause before their meals as adults and say, "I'm grateful that my mother taught me how to be grateful."

Grow a Gratitude Garden

I remember the day I met a young mama named Sandra at a playground. Sandra was a recently divorced single mom with four children and a limited income. We were chatting, and I was talking my typical organic talk. She looked at me wistfully and said, "I wish I could afford to feed my kids organic food and all that—but it's simply not my reality right now. If I have a choice between a two-dollar red pepper and four peppers for two dollars, I'm going to go with the one I can afford. I have four kids I'm trying to feed here."

I felt such compassion for this honest mama who was trying to do the best she could for her kids, and I know she's not alone. It's not just single mamas with four kids who are feeling the pinch these days—it's most of us. Organic food is expensive (although the prices are going down as demand goes up and farmers' markets often have organic produce at bargain prices), but what would you say to twenty, thirty, forty, or more organic red peppers for two dollars?

If you have a home with a little yard or even a porch, be filled with gratitude—because that means you can grow a garden!

Just as they have a natural fondness for animals, children have a natural affinity for the earth. They love putting their hands in the dirt and watching things grow. What better way to explore organic foods than growing your own garden? Even a tiny plot can grow lettuce, carrots, radishes, and other ingredients for a salad garden. A slightly larger plot could grow a salsa garden full of tomatoes, bell peppers, hot peppers, cilantro, and garlic.

If you have more space, you could also try growing strawberries, berry bushes, an apple tree, or grapevines. Larger plots could accommodate

---

Composting 101

You could start a compost pile and add compost to your garden twice a year. A little pile in an out-of-the-way corner of the yard can house your grass clippings, dead leaves, and all your nonanimal food scraps, from carrot peelings to avocado shells. A little bit of fencing or even chicken wire can keep the pile from spreading and keep pests out. Mix it up with a shovel every so often, water it when it gets dry, and at the beginning of every planting season, you've got black gold to nourish your garden.

Shovel it into the garden and mix it all up, and then watch your gorgeous organic veggies thrive. It's all the fertilizer you'll ever need, and you made it (with a little help from Mother Nature).

---

pumpkins, zucchini, watermelons, or butternut squash. Depending on your climate, you could try growing broccoli, cauliflower, eggplants, or artichokes. I know one organic papa who constructed teepee shapes out a few long wooden poles, one for each of his three children. He grew beans around the poles that climbed up and formed leafy green enclosures. The children loved to go inside their teepees in the summer to hide and pluck beans from the vines and have quiet time, or let their friends inside for secrets and giggling.

If you get excited about organic gardening, your child will, too, and it will be not only a foundation of good nutrition but a natural, empowering experience he'll always remember: *I grew my own food.*

Let your child help decide what sort of garden you should grow together. Gardening can be such a creative pursuit. Grow peas along the fence, grow beans on a trellis, plant strawberries in a sunny corner. Children are more likely to try eating vegetables such as tomatoes, bell peppers, green onions, carrots, peas, and green beans, if they have helped to grow them and harvest them. A child plucking peas out of a pod from a vine or cherry tomatoes from a tomato plant taller than she is and eating the fresh raw organic vegetables right there in your own backyard is a beautiful and inspiring sight.

Selfless Acts

As a parent, it's natural to want to help your kids learn to look out for themselves, but many children are naturally selfless. Encouraging this impulse will reinforce to your children that their natural impulses are on target. Some children naturally want to share, or even give their things away. I've actually seen parents discourage this natural impulse, saying things like, "Don't just give your things away!" or "Keep that for yourself!" or "That child doesn't deserve any help!" It breaks my heart to see that. Of course, a child must be guided away from being wasteful or giving away something she doesn't realize is too valuable or that the family needs, but the impulse itself should never be quashed.

Selflessness is a true spiritual gift, and a selfless act doesn't always have to be grand to be meaningful. It can be quite small—and frequent. Reinforce random selfless acts of kindness you see in your child, such as sharing a toy or a treat without being asked or making another child feel better when she is down. Also watch for empathy—when you notice that your child notices the pain or suffering of another, give her a hug and tell her she has a big heart. Because she does—and it's beautiful.

When children get involved in choosing seeds, planting them, and watching them grow, when they help weed and water and finally harvest the food for their own meal, they understand on a completely new level where and how food begins.

Even if you don't have a spot for an organic garden, you can grow herbs and certain vegetables such as tomatoes, peppers, green onions, or salad greens, in containers on your patio or even in a window box. It's a lesson in life, and a study on how nature provides for us, if we nurture it instead of destroying it. It's a beginning—and it will plant seeds of a different kind inside your child: seeds of hope and understanding and reverence.

Sandra's gratitude garden was a big success, and she became an eager and enthusiastic amateur gardener. Her children thought the garden was fun, too, especially since each one got a stone to paint. Four stones sat in that garden, each with a child's name, each a reminder that there is always a way to live a more organic life.

And when you harvest what you've grown with the help of nature and Mother Earth? Please, Mamas—give thanks.

Gratitude Vision Boards, Kid Edition

Most kids are visually oriented, and love to make and build things. Whether or not you made your own vision board (which I encouraged you to do in Chapter 8), try this fun project with your children.

The best way for this project to be successful is to get right down to business. Don't spend time explaining too much first (unless your child is more comfortable with that approach). Get right to the fun. Break out the old magazines, scissors, glue sticks, and poster boards. Encourage the kids to flip through the magazines and find things that show what they love that they already have in their lives—children tend to gravitate toward things they want, and you don't have to tell them they are wrong or can't include the picture of that great new toy on their vision boards. However, encourage them to also include things they love that they are thankful for—pictures of trees, perhaps, or the beach, pictures of families, animals in nature, pets, houses, cars, good food, friends having fun, playgrounds, amusement parks.

You could also include photos of your own family (print them out on an inkjet printer from your computer), pets, and adventures, such as fam-

Organic Voices

Through [the yoga principle of] Aparigraha, or non-greediness, we learn to be more satisfied with what we have and thankful for the abundance in our lives. We remember the blessing of our breath, the endless gifts of Mother Nature, and the pure joy of simply being alive and having the consciousness to be aware of it.

—*Bhava Ram,*
from *The 8 Limbs of Yoga*

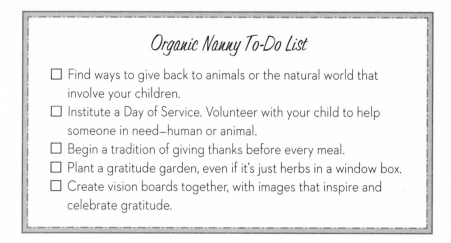

Organic Nanny To-Do List

☐ Find ways to give back to animals or the natural world that involve your children.
☐ Institute a Day of Service. Volunteer with your child to help someone in need—human or animal.
☐ Begin a tradition of giving thanks before every meal.
☐ Plant a gratitude garden, even if it's just herbs in a window box.
☐ Create vision boards together, with images that inspire and celebrate gratitude.

ily vacations, or let the children draw their own versions of these family members and adventures.

Make the board happy, joyful, cheery. Let her decorate it with glitter pens and stickers and anything else that makes her smile. When she is done, hang it in her room. The board will be a wonderful sparkly reminder of all she already has in her life—an inspiration and an invitation to live with an attitude of gratitude.

CHAPTER TWELVE

Listen from the Heart

You know more than you think you do.

—*Dr. Benjamin Spock*

*P*rior to the birth of their first son, Tucker, Laura and Mark thought they had it all figured out. They would often talk about the behavior of other people's children, knowingly conferring with each other and agreeing that no child of theirs would ever act like *that*. They had heard that babies shouldn't be coddled, toddlers needed discipline, children needed a strict schedule, and any child who learns that it is okay to inconvenience an adult will turn out to be spoiled rotten. All that made sense to them.

And all that changed after Tucker was born. Suddenly, with a newborn infant in her arms and at her breast, Laura didn't have the heart to let Tucker "cry it out." Her instinct told her to pick him up and hold him against her heart. Their carefully constructed schedules soon fell apart because sometimes Tucker was genuinely hungry before the scheduled mealtime, and sometimes he wasn't yet ready to eat when the metaphorical dinner bell rang. At night, nursing became easier with Tucker sleeping beside his mama. During the day, Laura felt compelled to carry Tucker in a sling instead of putting him in a playpen. It just felt right to her.

As he grew, Tucker became a round, happy baby with bright intelligent eyes. He was ultimately curious, and Mark also found that he didn't have the heart to tell his young son no or to "stop that" or "stop bothering me." He, too, found that although schedules sometimes worked, at other times the rules needed a bit of bending. He found he liked to be "inconvenienced" if it meant spending more time with his son and watching the miracle of a child learning about the world for the first time. His instinct told him to be with Tucker—that his child was more important than checking his e-mail.

When I came to help Mark and Laura, I could see what was happening, and I could see they were confused—they felt a little bit guilty that they hadn't adhered to their original plans for raising their child. I immediately did what I could to reinforce what they were doing, and I told them that in my experience, more time and physical contact and intuitive responding to a child's genuine needs in the moment results in a closer, more bonded family. Laura told me she was so relieved to hear that her instincts really were on target!

Intuition is something we all have, but learning to listen to it and acknowledge it and follow it is a skill. I call it listening from the heart, because that is what Tata called it, but it's intuition, pure and simple. It is that inner feeling that tells you exactly what your children really need, even when a book or a relative or a supposedly more experienced parent tells you differently. It is the impulse that urges you to pick up a baby when he cries, and to know when he just needs time to fall asleep on his own. It is that feeling you have when you just know something is wrong with your child, or that she is keeping a secret from you, or that she really needs to talk, or really needs time alone. It is one of the tools you get as a mother, and it's a tool you should use, perhaps more than you are using it now. Every family is unique, and every child is a precious treasure, unlike any other. You can apply, all day long, rules that other people have made, but at the end of the day, the way you interact with your children isn't about rules—not even the ones I've included in this book. It's about a parent's instinct.

In this last chapter, I want to empower you and inspire you to recognize that nobody knows your child the way you do. Learning to trust your own maternal instincts is the best thing you can do for your child. This chapter is about what you know, and about what your child knows, too.

How to Listen from the Heart

Listening from the heart is listening with all your senses. You listen with your ears, of course, but you also observe with your eyes. You feel with your hands. You sense certain energies. It is holistic listening.

When your child is upset, angry, sad, rebellious, or even when he says he is feeling sick, the first and most important thing you can do as a parent is to listen from the heart. The observant person can learn much more from the way a child expresses herself than by just the words.

I learned this skill from Tata, who always paid attention to the details people thought were extraneous but that they just happened to mention. She'd discover, for instance, that Miguel's wife was a very demanding woman, or that Consuela had been the family breadwinner since her husband lost his job. No wonder Miguel's head hurt—he felt beaten down all the time. No wonder Consuela had a backache. She felt as if she was carrying the weight of the world on her shoulders!

Tata heard the strain in the mama's voice when the child had a sore throat; she looked at the candy clutched in the fist of the hyperactive toddler; she observed the shoes of the little boy with the sore knees, or listened to the story of his long, hard walk home past a gauntlet of children who teased him.

Tata saw beyond a symptom and into the cause. You can, too.

Listening is the key to knowing how to help, support, and nurture your child in a way that suits her unique character. You may not always hear the answer or know what to do, but the more you listen without judgment, the more you will know, and knowledge will help you to make the best decision or say the right thing.

But listening can be surprisingly difficult. As parents, we are so prone to jumping in, interrupting, drawing conclusions, or thinking we already understand the situation. How often do you interrupt your child, or take something from her hand to do it for her more quickly, or tell her she doesn't really feel the way she says she feels? To be able to listen from the heart, this kind of reaction must stop first.

Here's an example of some typical exchanges I've heard between mother and child:

"Mom, I'm hungry." "No, you're not; you just ate."

"Mom, I'm not tired yet." "Yes, you are; it's past your bedtime."

"Mom, I think I'm sick." "No, you're not; you just don't want to go to school."

I hear parents do this all the time, and most of the time, I don't think they realize what they are doing. Of course parents would never want to undermine their child's self-confidence or sense of his own body and mind, but that's exactly what you are doing when you deny your child's truth. It's difficult to honor who a child is in any given moment, but it's absolutely essential if you are going to hone your intuition. You have to face the actual situation, not the one you wish was true.

When a child hears, over and over, that what he is feeling is not really what he is feeling, then he will learn not to trust himself. If he consistently learns that you can do things better than he can, he'll stop trying to do things for himself. If he learns that what he is saying isn't that important, he'll stop telling you things. He will lose touch with his own body and own emotions and own capabilities. He will look to others for validation, or even for others to tell him what to think and feel!

This is why, before you do anything else, you must first practice accepting that your child needs to learn to express himself and must learn to trust himself. Get out of the way.

For example, here are some alternative responses that will get you more information, rather than shutting down the source of information:

"Mom, I'm hungry." You say: "Help yourself to fruit or the bowl of veggies in the refrigerator—otherwise, we will be having a meal soon," or "That's unusual, since you ate not long ago. Are you bored? I can give you something to do."

If your child really has eaten enough, maybe she is actually trying to express a desire for something else, but the only way she knows how to describe it is by saying she is hungry. Listen for clues. Is she hungry for attention? For validation?

She may tell you she doesn't even know what she wants to eat, and that will be an opportunity for you to suggest some other activity—maybe something the two of you could do together. If she thinks she is hungry just because she is bored or lonely, you can fill her up without additional food. Giving her more food when what she really wanted was more time with you will only fuel her misguided body awareness and teach her to rely on food for comfort instead of human companionship. "I'm hungry" might just mean, "Sit down and talk to me."

Now, what about this one:

"Mom, I'm not tired yet." You say: "I know that it's hard to settle down for bed sometimes. Let's read a book first," or "It's getting late. Let's have a snack and work on getting sleepy."

Banishing your child to a dark room without getting to the bottom of why he thinks he doesn't want to go to bed yet is counterproductive and could just make sleep issues worse. Instead, acknowledge how he feels and try to help. Sleep is important, and you can explain this and tell him that even if he just lies in bed and rests, he is still getting the benefits of sleep. Does he need a stuffed animal friend? A nightlight? A lullaby?

Sometimes "I'm not tired yet" also really means, "Sit down and talk to me."

And finally, what about this one:

"Mom, I think I'm sick." You say: "Oh, that's not good! Tell me more about how you feel."

When a child says she is sick, it is a sure sign that something is going on, even if it's not an actual illness (or maybe it really is). Maybe she really is sick of school or having trouble with friends, or maybe she is nervous about something and she is interpreting that uncomfortable feeling as illness. Or, she might really be feeling the first signs of a cold or some other disease. She may not know, and she needs you to help her unpuzzle the feeling.

Asking for more information is the first step. Investigate any specific complaints, or if you don't hear any, then ask about what's coming. "What are you doing in school today? Are you nervous about something? How are things with your friends?" You may not get a direct answer, but watch for clues—how she talks, where she looks, how she uses her hands—and listen, listen, listen. Does she just need a little bit of attention, or does her forehead really feel warm?

Tata taught me that many times, symptoms are actually symbolic clues to a root cause: the headache in response to nagging, the back pain in response to excessive responsibility, fevers when the home environment is too "hot" and stressful, sore throats when there is too much yelling or communication is being repressed, stomachaches due to dread or fear, constipation due to holding in feelings, diarrhea due to a lack of feeling in control.

Organic Voices

The first duty of love is to listen.
—*Paul Tillich*

But sometimes, the answer is even simpler: a healthy diet and lifestyle builds a healthy body and immune system. Not every complaint is a metaphor! Sometimes, your child means quite literally what he says, such as that a tummy or throat hurts, or something itches or stings or aches. Unhealthy food, lack of exercise, lack of fresh air, and too much stress can throw a wrench in the body's workings and things can start to fall apart, or you may never know why somebody caught a bug. Sometimes it just happens—someone sneezes at school and your child inhales a virus. Learn everything you can by opening your ears and your eyes and your heart. Only then can you figure out what to do about it.

Sometimes, the most difficult part of listening from the heart is truly believing that you know best. Do you typically discount that small voice inside you that tells you what you already know? Do you wait for proof, or do you act on instinct? Sometimes, listening from the heart means listening to yourself, and acting on your feelings instead of the facts. When you become a mother, you are endowed with the gift of a special brand of highly attuned intuition that applies specifically to your own children. Mamas, I encourage you to trust that voice.

Of course, there is a difference between excessive worrying and actual intuition, and sometimes these can be hard to distinguish, but worrying feels anxious and obsessive. You will run through long lists in your head of what could be wrong or what might happen. Intuition comes from a deeper, calmer place. Sometimes, all it takes to find it and hear it is to sit quietly for a few moments and breathe deeply and focus very clearly on a single question, such as, "Why is my child sad?" or "What should I do about this problem?" and the answer will come to you, clear as a bell. Remember how I encouraged you to practice meditation in the Phenomenal Mamas chapter? This is an excellent way to refine, clarify, and turn up the volume on your intuition. It's in there, I promise. All you have to do is listen.

About Discipline

Up until this point, you may have a feeling that this chapter is pretty touchy-feely, that all children are perfect angels if we only treat them kindly, and that parenting is pretty easy if we just lay off a little.

We all know that's not true.

Your children are a part of you, but they are also their own little people, unique individuals with desires and aversions and strong opinions, even as infants. Sometimes, despite your best efforts, your child is going to misbehave: do something you very clearly told him not to do, or take a dangerous risk, or talk back, or do something unkind to a sibling or another child at school.

So what do you do when your child is "naughty"?

Some parents believe that if they are too responsive to a child's needs, that means the child can get away with anything, but nothing could be further from the truth. In fact, it's the opposite. The more in tune you are to your child's individual needs, the more you will discover where he needs freedom and where he needs boundaries. All children need both.

I'm not a fan of the word *discipline*, because it sounds punitive or even violent, and no matter what a child does, I don't think any sort of violence is ever warranted, not even a spanking. However, I am a strong proponent of *boundaries*.

Behavior problems are complex, and they require parental intuition to know how to handle them. Sometimes, they even require professional intervention, in the form of a family therapist or counselor. In most cases, however, behavior problems aren't chronic. They just happen sometimes, and they can stem from so many causes—poor health, poor nutrition, or a lack of supervision or guidance or knowledge or even exercise! They can also be caused by children's natural exploration of the world, or desire to see how much they can do without your intervention. Often, behavior problems are calls for more attention from you. Sometimes they are just a matter of children working out how to live in the world. A child may be experimenting with his own personality and figuring out what works and what doesn't or who he wants to be. Some "naughtiness" isn't really naughtiness at all. It's more a matter of a child's doing something a parent just doesn't like, or that becomes inconvenient.

Each of these scenarios calls for a different kind of response, but do you spank a child for getting poor nutrition? Of course not! You give him better food. In my experience, bad behavior is not a reason to spank a child either. It's a reason to give him something she needs, whether that is a restriction, a responsibility, a consequence, or a change in routine. None of those responses call for anger or violence on the part of the responsible adult.

But how do you know what to do and when? This is where your intuition comes into play. That involves some work. You have to talk to your child, ask him why he did what he did, what he was thinking or feeling—find out as much as you can. Look to yourself. Were you missing something? Did you fail to provide some sort of guidance or restriction? If not, why did your child blatantly disregard your rule? What would be an appropriate consequence? Does your child require a new rule, or a reaffirmation of an old rule, or a new restriction based on his inability to follow the less restrictive environment?

Of course, I cannot tell you what to do because I am not the parent of your child, but I urge you to take responsibility for your child's misbehavior, not by blaming yourself for it, but in a sort of detective role. Get to the bottom of it. Talk it out with another adult. Then act.

Most important, remain calm. Any sort of guidance or reaction from you will be much more powerful and much less frightening if you don't lose it in front of your child. If your emotions are getting out of control, give yourself a time-out to think about what you are doing before you act. Never punish out of anger. Wait, breathe, and let your heart lead you by using all your senses to figure out what happened.

To help guide you, I've written a few rules for *you* that I believe will help you better deal with misbehavior from your child. Try these and see which ones work in your family.

Good Behavior Rules for Parents

1. No time-outs for children.

When Tucker became a toddler, he was into everything, and sometimes his behavior wore on his parents' patience. When I came to help them, they were surprised to learn that I didn't approve of time-outs, and that not only would I not be giving Tucker any time-outs, but I suggested they refrain from the practice, too. I told them to stay with Tucker when he misbehaved, rather than banishing him. This is different than rewarding misbehavior. Instead, you are listening, gathering information.

You can stay with a toddler who is having a tantrum, without feeding into the energy of the tantrum. Tantrums are often calls for attention. Removing the child and yourself from a public situation is appropriate, but staying with the child and watching closely for signs of what's really causing the distress, can be informative . . . and even puzzling to the child. Why aren't you screaming back? What are you looking at? I've seen a listening mama diffuse a tantrum just by watching her child with interest as he kicked and screamed. He suddenly sat up, perhaps recognizing that she was giving him her full, calm attention, and asked if she would go to the park with him.

Tucker's parents agreed to try my method for a while, and they were amazed by how quickly Tucker responded. Within a few days, he was behaving more as they wished. His mama told me, "It really works! When I stay with him and tune in to why he is doing something I don't like, suddenly it becomes obvious to me, and I can redirect him or distract him or give him something better to do. No tantrums—when I stay with him, he's happy to do something else."

When you don't send a child away from the family in shame, you are forced to face the problem instead of shove it away. Sending children away doesn't help them understand that they should not do something. It just gets them away from you for a few minutes. Telling them directly that they are not allowed to behave the way they are behaving and then immediately redirecting their focus to something else works much better.

My only exception to the no time-outs rule is that time-out *you* may need. When you need one, by all means, take it! This also provides a good model for your children. As they get older, many children learn to leave a situation when it becomes too emotional or unproductive. They give themselves a time-out and are then better able to diffuse their own anger. Sometimes a few minutes alone to calm down will make all the difference in the world to anyone who is upset.

2. No hand-slapping.

As much as you may feel the urge to slap away a curious little hand reaching for a forbidden whatever-it-is, this is my second rule for parents: No hand-slapping! (And no slapping anything else, either.) According to Maria Montessori, children's hands are a natural extension of their mind. Children explore the world with their hands. Slapping those hands is like slapping your children's natural curiosity, or telling them their impulse to reach out and discover the world is wrong and bad. Of course we don't want to send that message to our children!

Organic Voices

If we truly want peace in the world, let us begin by loving one another in our own families.

—*Mother Teresa*

If it's a matter of preventing injury, you can stop a child's hand without slapping it. Besides, any kind of hitting sends the message that hitting is a way to deal with a problem. That's another message I don't believe you want to send your child. Hold your child's hand, pick him up, redirect him, tell him no. But don't slap.

3. Reward good behavior.

It's so easy to focus on bad behavior and it's so easy to let good behavior slide by unnoticed. Bad behavior is annoying at best, and potentially dangerous. Good behavior is easy.

However, research shows that when children are rewarded for good behavior instead of punished for bad behavior, they are more motivated to behave well. Children want good things—especially your undivided attention. Give it to your child when he is doing what you want, even if it means he is sitting quietly and patiently waiting for you to get off the phone. Get off the phone and sit with him for a while! He's being good and he needs to know what that means. Otherwise, all he will know is how not to be bad.

4. Acknowledge how your child feels, even if you don't like how she feels.

Children brought up to believe their feelings are valid and they are capable and loveable and worth listening to have much higher self-esteem and, consequently, higher achievement than do children who grow up believing they are irresponsible or unlikable, that their feelings aren't valid, or they are not worth listening to. You may not realize it, but whenever you undermine a child's feelings, you send a message that he can't trust himself. Bite your tongue when you are tempted to criticize, and just listen. Repeat back how your child feels.

For example, instead of saying, "You shouldn't yell at your brother; he's only three!" you could say, "I can see that you are very angry when your brother bothers you."

This simple approach opens up a whole new world to a child: He isn't naughty! He's just angry, and you are willing to help him deal with those strong feelings. Once he knows you are really listening, he will be more likely to express to you what he is really feeling, rather than feeling powerless or ashamed.

5. It's about the situation, not the child.

Every behavior problem is a problem with a situation, not a problem with the child herself. Let your language reflect this. Instead of, "Get your coat—you always forget things!" you can say, "Your coat needs to go to school with you."

6. Heal with laughter.

Oh, Mamas, how can I emphasize enough to you the importance of a life and a household full of laughter? Especially when the air is tense, when your child is screaming, when you feel like your head is going to explode, remember this: You have two options. You can choose to make it worse, or you can choose to make it better.

You won't always say the right thing, and changing your approach to discipline takes time. You can't just snap your fingers and make all your knee-jerk responses disappear. However, when the pressure mounts, one of the best ways I know to make it better is to diffuse the situation with laughter. Let your life be fun! Give yourself permission to have fun. Make a silly joke. Make a funny face. Distract your screaming child with a goofy gesture. After a long day, watch a funny movie. Read a funny book. Collect jokes. Giggle. Tickle (respectfully). Laugh. Joy is made out of laughter, and laughter heals like nothing else I know. So when in doubt, when you just don't know what else to do, laugh. It's natural to get angry and it's natural to be sad sometimes, but if you can learn to laugh more in your life, those negative feelings won't last for long.

Organic Voices

A smile starts on the lips, a grin spreads to the eyes, a chuckle comes from the belly, but a good laugh bursts forth from the soul. Overflows, and bubbles all around.

—*Carolyn Birmingham*

Remembering these six rules will help you gently teach yourself how to step back and listen from the heart instead of being reactive in a way that doesn't help. Think back on how you felt as a child when someone yelled at you or told you that you were bad or slapped your hand or said you didn't really feel what you felt. Helpless? Powerless? Furious? Ashamed? Those are not productive feelings in a child. They do not promote the kind of inner strength and pride you want for your child.

Listening, laughing, and loving won't spoil your child. Positive interactions show respect. In fact, you can deal with anybody this way. When you stop yelling and punishing and you start listening and smiling, you will feel an immense relief and inner calm, and suddenly, the world makes more sense. Try it, the next time you feel overwhelmed. Then sit down with your children and listen.

Listen to Yourself

Finally, one of the things I often notice when I come to help a new family is that the parents are very good at listening to their child—but not so good at listening to themselves. Every family is unique and different, and nobody else's rules need apply to your family.

When I first met Peter and Helena on a Saturday afternoon in New York City's Central Park, they had been married only two years. They had just had a brand-new baby, and Helena was coming to the end of her maternity leave. As I chatted with them, I noticed how much Helena talked about her job and how much Peter talked about baby Howard.

Both Peter and Helena had stressful jobs. They were a true New York power couple with packed schedules, so maternity leave had been an unusually calm time for them, despite the demands of an infant. Now they were trying to figure out what to do because Helena was ready to go back to work.

Organic Voices

The greatest deficit in America isn't the trade deficit. It's the attention deficit of our children. The average child gets 14 minutes of attention a day from each of his parents. So the greatest thing you can give a kid is time spent listening to him or her.

—Jack Canfield

Helena was torn—of course she loved her baby and wanted to be a good mother, but she knew that she was already missing out on career opportunities at the office. She couldn't imagine not working.

Pete, on the other hand, seemed less thrilled about his corporate job. They weren't comfortable with hiring someone else to raise their child.

One afternoon, after listening to them, I said, "Why can't Pete stay home with baby Howard?"

I remember the way that Pete and Helena stared at each other, as if they had never even considered this possibility. I pointed out to them how many fathers were right there in the park with young children, and I could see a light go on in Pete's eyes.

Pete left his corporate job to stay home and take care of his son and their new adopted dog, Duke, whom they rescued from the ASPCA. I would see him occasionally, at the farmers' market or the playground, and he looked as happy as I've ever seen a papa look. Soon after, Pete started a blog about his experiences as a stay-at-home dad. He detailed his adventures with his son, building tent houses in the living room, making their own Halloween costumes, and documenting his son's childhood with a digital camera. Meanwhile, Helena was soon promoted and the family was easily able to live off of her newly increased salary. Everyone was happy.

This is just one example of finding a way to be a family that works for you, even if it isn't what other people might consider "normal." Who defines *normal*, anyway? Listen to your own needs and the needs of every member in your family, and you can reclaim control over what and who you want to be in the world. It's nobody else's business what's right for you. Best of all, your children will learn from you how to follow their own heart, their own intuition, and their instincts about what is right and wrong. This is what it all comes down to in the end: teaching your children how to live their own lives and be fulfilled.

Mamas, life is short and precious. We only have a small amount of time with our children before they become adults with children of their own. What you do now, every moment matters, and I don't want you to miss any of it. Instead, I want you to make the most of it.

Charles Swindoll once wrote, "Each day of our lives we make deposits in the memory banks of our children." Invest in those deposits, and watch your children bloom. When you build a healthy life for your children, and then let yourself enjoy it by listening and cherishing every moment with your very special family, you are *living*. Feed them well, teach them reverence for life, encourage their bodies to heal naturally, foster in them appreciation for what they have, steer them away from screens and into nature, guide them toward a life of gratitude and the habit of service, and by all means, take care of yourself, too. Most important of all, listen to your heart and act on its message. This is the organic way. This is the natural way. And this is the way I believe children and parents were meant to live: in a beautiful harmony with each other and the world. You

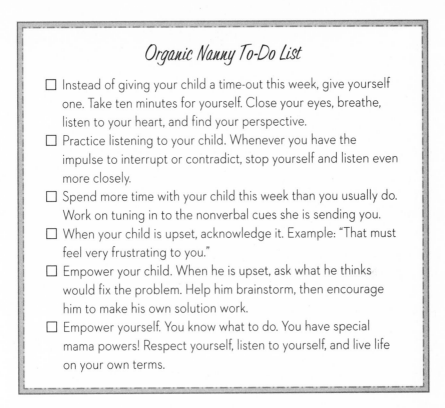

Organic Nanny To-Do List

☐ Instead of giving your child a time-out this week, give yourself one. Take ten minutes for yourself. Close your eyes, breathe, listen to your heart, and find your perspective.

☐ Practice listening to your child. Whenever you have the impulse to interrupt or contradict, stop yourself and listen even more closely.

☐ Spend more time with your child this week than you usually do. Work on tuning in to the nonverbal cues she is sending you.

☐ When your child is upset, acknowledge it. Example: "That must feel very frustrating to you."

☐ Empower your child. When he is upset, ask what he thinks would fix the problem. Help him brainstorm, then encourage him to make his own solution work.

☐ Empower yourself. You know what to do. You have special mama powers! Respect yourself, listen to yourself, and live life on your own terms.

are building a better childhood for your children, and fostering a better Earth for all children.

All my love and all my heart to you, organic Mamas and Papas. May your family be blessed and filled with light, and may you feel a deep connection with all life and know that you belong here.

Appendix One

Organic Nanny Kid-Friendly Recipes

These are just a handful of my favorite ideas and recipes, tested on a group of twelve children and eight mamas. We discovered that the kids most preferred simple foods, vegetables in "hidden" form, and sweet and salty tastes. We sure had fun cooking and eating together, and I hope you will have just as much fun trying our creative concoctions. I also want to thank Chef Gabrielle Mittelstaedt, former head chef of the much-loved Peaceful Planet restaurant in Nashville, for pointing this book in the yummiest direction.

Beverages

Organic Nanny Juice

Serves 1 child. Can be doubled, tripled, or more.
This easy, adaptable juice can be made with any fruits and vegetables. Keep trying different combinations to discover new family favorites.

    1 juicy orchard fruit, such as a ripe apple, pear, or peach (before
        juicing, core the apple or pear, or remove the pit from the
        peach)
    1 orange, cut into sections
    1 carrot, trimmed and scrubbed (removes bitterness)

Run everything through the juicer. Serve immediately.

Smoothie "Medicine"

A great use for smoothies is to provide extra nutrition when a child is sick. Sick children often don't want to eat, but they will drink something. Smoothies can also help with constipation because the fiber in the fruit softens the bowels. Add flaxseed oil to a bedtime smoothie for a gentle overnight laxative effect—no cramps, no drugs. Add protein powder and/or a spoonful of almond butter to a morning smoothie for a dose of protein to keep your child nourished and energetic throughout the day. For a child who needs to put on a little bit of weight, nut butters make an excellent addition to smoothies.

As your child gets more accustomed to fresh juice, try adding other fruit and vegetables. Let your child help with the juice experiments. What juice could she create and name after herself? Some produce to try (peel all fruit with thick, inedible skins):

- Apricot
- Avocado
- Beet
- Celery
- Grapes
- Grapefruit
- Kiwi
- Leafy greens—add a single large leaf of kale, chard, collard greens, or a romaine romaine lettuce leaf
- Mango
- Papaya
- Pineapple
- Plum
- Steamed veggies, such as broccoli, green beans, or peas
- Tomato

Organic Nanny Smoothie _____

Serves 1 child (or double the recipe and you can share)
This is the classic smoothie I always make, although I vary it according to each child's taste, and I always start with fewer greens and work up to more.

Juice from 1/2 lemon
1/2 fresh or frozen ripe banana (frozen makes a creamier-textured smoothie)
1/2 cup fresh or frozen brightly colored berries (e.g., blueberries or strawberries, or a combination)
1 fresh leaf kale, chard, or romaine lettuce (or less than 1 leaf at first)
1 teaspoon fresh, refrigerated flaxseed oil (start with less if your child can taste it)
1 tablespoon real maple syrup (more or less, depending on your child's taste)
4 ice cubes

Optional:
1 scoop vanilla or chocolate protein powder (look for one with vitamin B_{12} added)

Puree everything in a blender until well combined. If the smoothie is too thick, add a little bit of purified water or nondairy milk, such as rice or almond milk. Serve immediately—with or without a spoon!

Once your child has gotten into the juice-and-smoothie habit, get creative together. Very gradually increase the proportion of leafy greens to fruit (ideally you will work up to half greens, half fruit), but keep it yummy. If your child doesn't like it, back off the green stuff a bit. Remember, never force your child to eat! Better to throw away a bad batch of juice or smoothie than to create tension and negative feelings about food.

Special additions that can make the smoothie even sweeter:

- 1 teaspoon unsweetened cocoa powder or raw cacao nibs
- Pinch of cinnamon
- Drop of vanilla extract or other flavored extract

Back-to-Basics Smoothie

If your child is resistant to smoothies, start with an even simpler recipe: Blend a frozen banana or 1 cup of frozen berries with just enough nondairy milk (e.g., rice or almond milk) to make a sweet, ice-creamy treat. Then, introduce new ingredients gradually, one at a time. There is no hurry.

- 1 teaspoon ground flaxseed or flaxseed oil
- 1 teaspoon raw wheat germ
- 1 tablespoon nut (e.g., almond or cashew) or peanut butter
- Any other fresh or frozen fruit you happen to have on hand

Purple Power Smoothie

Serves 2

This brilliant purple smoothie tastes so fruity, they'll never know it contains leafy greens—not to mention tons of antioxidants, flavonoids, and resveratrol, which have anticancer, anti-inflammatory, and antiallergic effects, and may also protect against future heart disease. Talk about purple power!

1 cup frozen blueberries
1/2 cup organic grape juice
1 scoop protein powder (e.g., brown rice or soy protein)
1 leaf kale or romaine lettuce

Combine all the ingredients in a blender and blend until completely smooth. Serve immediately.

Secret Agent Smoothie

Serves 2

I've had to use a little espionage to get some of my clients' children to try smoothies. This one has always done the trick. Of course, the vegetables are the secret agents, but kids just love the name. It sounds like they know something the grown-ups don't!

1 cup any berries (fresh or frozen)
1 fresh leaf kale, chard, or romaine lettuce (or less than 1 leaf at first)
1 cup almond milk
1 scoop protein powder (I prefer a vegetable source, e.g., brown rice
   or soy protein)
1 tablespoon real maple syrup
1/4 teaspoon ground cinnamon
4 ice cubes

Puree everything in a blender until well combined. Serve immediately—with or without a spoon!

Orange-Strawberry Smoothie
Serves 2

A delicious sweet breakfast treat, and an excellent reason to keep frozen strawberries in your freezer at all times. This smoothie is rich in vitamin C, fiber, and antioxidants.

1 cup frozen strawberries
1/2 cup orange juice
1/2 cup vanilla-flavored or plain rice or almond milk
1 tablespoon real maple syrup (or agave syrup, for an even sweeter
   smoothie)

Combine all the ingredients in a blender. Blend until thick and creamy. Pour into glasses or cups and enjoy immediately.

Breakfast

Blueberry Pancakes with Strawberry Sauce
Serves 4

These sweet, fruity, juicy pancakes are a real treat for a weekend breakfast. Who wouldn't love to wake up to pancakes on a Saturday morning? Topped with strawberry sauce, these pancakes are especially vitamin rich and brimming with antioxidants.

1 1/2 cups organic whole wheat pastry flour

1/2 cup organic oat flour (or blend organic oats in a blender to
    create flour)

1 tablespoon baking powder

1 teaspoon ground cinnamon

1/2 teaspoon salt

2 cups rice or almond milk

2 tablespoons canola oil

1 tablespoon real maple syrup

1 teaspoon vanilla extract

Cooking spray

1 cup fresh blueberries

Strawberry Sauce:

2 cups fresh sliced or frozen strawberries

1/2 cup organic orange, apple, cherry, or any other natural 100%
    fruit juice

1/2 cup real maple syrup

*In a large bowl with a spout (e.g., an 8-cup glass measure), combine
the flours, baking powder, cinnamon, and salt with a wire whisk.*

*In a separate bowl, combine milk, oil, maple syrup, and vanilla
extract with a wire whisk. Add the wet ingredients to the dry and
stir gently, until just combined. A few lumps remaining are fine. Set
aside to thicken.*

*Spray a griddle or large skillet with cooking spray and heat over
medium heat. While the pan is heating, start the strawberry sauce
by combining the strawberries and syrup in a large saucepan over
medium-high heat. Stir every minute or so until the mixture begins
to bubble. Lower the heat and simmer until the mixture is reduced
by half. Remove from the heat and set aside.*

*When the griddle is hot, give the pancake batter a final stir and
pour small pancakes (about 3 inches in diameter) onto the griddle.
Sprinkle each pancake with a few blueberries. Watch the pancakes*

carefully to prevent burning. When the edges bubble, gently flip them over. Depending on the size of your pan, you may need to make several batches. Wipe off and respray the griddle carefully between batches, and keep pancakes on a heat-proof plate in a warm oven (less than 300°F) until you are ready to serve them.

Serve the pancakes warm, drizzled with the strawberry syrup. Freeze leftover pancakes in resealable plastic bags in the freezer and reheat in a toaster or microwave. Store any leftover strawberry sauce in a glass jar with a lid in the refrigerator, for up to 1 week.

Fried Tofu Breakfast Sandwich

Serves 1. Can be doubled, tripled, or more.

Your homemade L.O.V.E. version of a fast-food drive-through breakfast. Fried tofu tastes remarkably like a fried egg in these sandwiches.

Toasted sesame or canola oil
1 (3-ounce) slice extra-firm tofu, drained and patted dry with paper
  towels
2 teaspoons soy sauce
1 whole wheat English muffin
1 teaspoon trans-fat-free, nondairy butter (e.g., Earth Balance)

Optional:
1 veggie sausage patty, cooked according to the package directions,
  and/or a fresh tomato slice

Heat a nonstick skillet over medium-high heat. Pour in and heat the sesame oil. Add the tofu slice over the sesame oil and sprinkle half the soy sauce on the top. Fry until one side is golden and crispy. Flip over, top with the remaining soy sauce, and fry until the second side is golden and crispy.

Toast the English muffin and butter it. Put the tofu on the bottom half of the English muffin, top with sausage patty and/or tomato slice, if using, then top with remaining muffin half. Serve warm.

L.O.V.E. Muffins _____

Makes 12 muffins

These bright, citrusy, sunshiny muffins are brimming with L.O.V.E.—and vitamin C and omega-3 fatty acids from the flaxseeds. What a happy way to start your morning!

   2 cups organic whole wheat pastry flour
   1/4 cup organic ground flaxseeds
   1 1/2 teaspoons baking powder
   1 teaspoon baking soda
   1 teaspoon ground cinnamon
   1/2 teaspoon salt
   1 cup vanilla-flavored almond or rice milk
   1/2 cup organic orange juice concentrate, thawed
   2 tablespoons real maple syrup
   1 tablespoon canola oil
   Juice and grated zest from 1 organic lemon
   1 cup organic dried cranberries or cherries (look for the naturally
      sweetened kind)

Preheat the oven to 375°F. In a large bowl, combine the flour, baking powder, baking soda, cinnamon, and salt, with a wire whisk.

In a separate bowl, combine the milk, orange juice concentrate, maple syrup, canola oil, and lemon juice and zest. Add the wet ingredients to the dry and stir just until combined. Stir in dried cranberries.

Put paper liners in a twelve-cup muffin pan. Pour the batter into the prepared pan, filling the cups no more than three-quarters full. Bake for 30 minutes, or until a toothpick inserted into the center of a muffin comes out clean. Let cool for at least 10 minutes. Serve warm or at room temperature.

The avocado is a superfood. Adding a little pureed hummus to this recipe provides protein. Adding cilantro provides vitamins A and C.

Dips, Sides, and Main Dishes

Simple Guacamole

Serves 2. Can be doubled, tripled, or more.
Rich avocados have a simple flavor many kids love.

    1 ripe avocado, halved and pitted
    1/2 teaspoon salt
    Juice from 1/2 fresh lime

Optional:
1 tablespoon minced fresh cilantro

Scoop the avocado flesh into a bowl. Add the salt and lime juice. Mash with a fork. Stir in the cilantro, if using. Serve immediately.

Hummus

Serves 4 to 6
Hummus can be expensive in the store, which is silly because it's so quick to make. Just break out the blender or food processor. Hummus is an excellent snack or meal because it is full of strength-building protein and iron.

    1 (15-ounce) can organic garbanzo beans (chickpeas), drained and
       rinsed
    1 tablespoon tahini (sesame butter) or peanut butter
    Juice from 1 lemon
    1/2 teaspoon salt
    Water, for thinning

Put all the ingredients, except the water, in a blender or food processor. Blend. If the hummus is too thick, add the water 1 tablespoon at a time until you reach the desired consistency (hummus can be thick for spreading, or a little thinner for dipping).

Cuban Salsa

Serves 4

A fruity take on salsa, this is rich with vitamin C.

1 mango, peeled and cubed
1/2 fresh pineapple, peeled and cubed
1/4 cup finely chopped fresh cilantro
1/2 teaspoon salt
Juice from 1 lime

Optional:
A bit of minced jalapeño pepper

Combine all the ingredients in a bowl. Cover and refrigerate for at least 30 minutes, or overnight. Enjoy in tacos (see page 236), with baked tortilla chips, or just eat it with a spoon.

Homemade French Fries

Serves 2. Can be doubled, tripled, or more.

These are easy, much better for your child than fast-food fries, and potatoes are high in vitamins B_6 and C, potassium, and fiber.

Olive oil cooking spray
1 large or two medium-size potatoes, any kind (baking, yellow, red, sweet)
1/2 teaspoon salt

Preheat the oven to 400°F. Spray a baking sheet with cooking spray. Scrub the potatoes, cut out any blemishes in the skin, peel if desired

*(it's not necessary if your child will eat the skin), and cut into French
fry shapes.*

*Spread the fries on the baking sheet with a rim. Line them up so
they do not touch one another. Spray with more cooking spray and
sprinkle with salt. Bake for 30 to 45 minutes, turning or stirring the
fries once after about 20 minutes, until the fries look golden brown
and crispy. Serve warm.*

Organic Nanny Mashed Potatoes

Serves 4

Old-time comfort food. Most kids love mashed potatoes.

> 4 medium-size white or yellow potatoes
> 1/2 cup nondairy milk
> 1/4 cup trans-fat-free nondairy butter (e.g., Earth Balance)
> 1 teaspoon salt

*Peel the potatoes and boil them in a large pot of salted water until
they are fork-tender, about 30 minutes. Drain them and put them in
a large bowl. Add the milk, butter, and salt. Mash with a potato
masher. For a smoother texture, beat with an electric beater on low
speed. Serve warm.*

Cuban Mashed Sweet Potatoes

Serves 4

So sweet, creamy, and enticing, these mashed sweet potatoes are easy for
toddlers to eat with a little spoon, and just as satisfying for teenagers, not to
mention everyone in between (grown-ups love them, too).

> 3 large or 4 small sweet potatoes or yams
> 1 tablespoon olive oil or nondairy nonhydrogenated margarine (e.g.,
> Earth Balance)
> 1 teaspoon ground cumin (optional; some children may prefer
> sweet potatoes plain)
> 1 teaspoon salt

Optional toppings:
Chopped pecans
Raisins
A bit of real maple syrup

Preheat the oven to 375°F. Scrub the sweet potatoes clean with a vegetable brush, then dry them. Prick each sweet potato a few times with a fork. Put them directly on the oven rack. Bake them for about 1 hour, or until they feel soft and squishy when lightly squeezed.

Remove them from the oven. When they are cool enough to handle, cut them open and scoop the potato pulp into a bowl. Add the oil, cumin, and salt. Stir until completely combined. Serve warm, with or without toppings.

Green Salad

Serves any number

This isn't really a recipe, but I want to talk about green salads. A lot of kids don't like greens, but they are so nutritious that it's a good idea to experiment with the best ways to make green salads appealing to your child. Make your own, switch it up, or ask your child for input.

Tear bright, crisp lettuce into bite-size pieces. Try bright, sweet lettuces such as buttercrunch, iceberg, and romaine. Drizzle with a favorite dressing (many kids like ranch or peanut dressing—look for bottled organic varieties such as Newman's Own or Annie's Naturals), sprinkle with peanuts and raisins, or make a face out of a leaf of lettuce by adding grape eyes, a cherry tomato nose, and a mouth made from a carrot curl or a strip of sweet red pepper.

Organic Nanny Tacos

Serves any number

Lots of healthy toppings in bowls on the table allow kids to assemble their own tacos. The ingredients in this list are just suggestions—include foods your child likes, and a few they haven't tried yet. The more vegetables you offer, the more likely your child is to try them—and reap all the nutritional benefits!

1 or 2 taco shells per person

Suggested toppings:

Black or refried beans

Veggie "crumbles" (resembles ground beef) or "chicken" (resembles chicken strips). Or, if you are still transitioning, try organic locally raised chicken cut into cubes or shreds.

Shredded lettuce

Chopped tomatoes

Chopped olives

Guacamole

Cuban Salsa (page 234)

Tofu Fingers

Serves 4 to 6

Easy to eat, easy to love! Tofu is rich in protein, one of the less processed forms of soy, and one or two servings of soy per day should be fine for most kids.

Cooking spray

1 pound extra-firm tofu, drained and patted dry with paper towels

2 tablespoons soy sauce

1/2 cup whole wheat pastry flour

1 tablespoon ground flaxseeds mixed with 1/4 cup water (or one organic egg, lightly beaten)

2 cups rice cereal (e.g., Rice Krispies, although I prefer the organic brown rice version)

Preheat the oven to 350°F. Spray a baking sheet with cooking spray.

Cut the block of tofu into sixteen long strips. Put them in a shallow bowl. Sprinkle with the soy sauce. Set aside.

Put the flour on a large plate. Place the flaxseed mixture in a shallow bowl. Put the cereal on another plate.

Take a strip of tofu, roll it in the flour, dip it in the flaxseed mixture, roll it in the cereal, then place it on the baking sheet. Repeat with all the strips.

Bake until crispy, about 40 minutes, turning the strips once with tongs. Serve warm.

Make-Your-Own Pizzas _____

Serves 4

This is such an easy and fun dinner for a party or just for the family, because everybody loves pizza, and every pizza is custom-made for individual tastes, picky or not.

> 4 individual-size pizza crusts
> 1 cup organic tomato sauce
> 1 teaspoon dried oregano

> *Everyone's favorite toppings, such as:*
> Sliced mushrooms
> Chopped tomatoes
> Green and red bell pepper strips
> Artichoke hearts
> Sliced olives
> Chopped onions
> Shredded veggie cheese (or real organic cheese, if transitioning)

> *Let everyone assemble his or her own pizza, then bake on baking sheets in a preheated 400°F oven until hot and bubbly.*

Pasta with Red Sauce _____

Serves 4

This simple red sauce contains "secret" veggies for powerful nutrition that your child won't even notice. An immersion blender is handy for pureeing this sauce, but a regular blender will work, too.

> 1 tablespoon olive oil
> 1 small onion, peeled and chopped
> 1 small zucchini, trimmed and grated
> 1 carrot, trimmed and grated
> 2 to 4 fresh kale leaves, chopped finely
> 2 garlic cloves, peeled and minced
> 1 (15-ounce) can organic tomato sauce

1 cup water or vegetable broth
1 (4-ounce) can organic tomato paste
1 teaspoon dried oregano
1/2 teaspoon dried thyme
1/2 teaspoon salt
8 to 12 ounces whole wheat pasta in your favorite shape

Heat the oil in a large sauté pan with a lid over medium-high heat. Add the onion, zucchini, carrot, kale, and garlic. Sauté the vegetables, stirring frequently, until they are soft and begin to turn golden, about 15 minutes.

When the vegetables start to brown, add the tomato sauce, water, tomato paste, herbs, and salt. Stir to combine. When the sauce begins to bubble, cover the pan and lower the heat to medium-low. Simmer for 1 hour. Turn off the heat and puree the sauce with an immersion blender, or transfer in batches to a blender and puree (be careful blending hot liquids—don't fill the blender more than half full).

About 20 minutes before the sauce is done, begin cooking the pasta according to the package directions. When the pasta is done, drain and divide it among four plates. Ladle the sauce over the pasta. Store any leftover sauce in the refrigerator for another easy pasta meal.

Whole-Grain Garlic Bread

Crusty garlic bread is mild and perfect for dipping in sauce—but kids can refuse to let it touch their sauce, too.

1 loaf whole-grain French or Italian bread (a long, thin loaf)
1/2 cup trans-fat-free, nondairy butter (e.g., Earth Balance)
1 teaspoon garlic powder (preferably in a shaker)

Preheat the oven to 375°F. Cut the loaf into 1-inch slices. Butter each slice and put the slices on a baking sheet. Sprinkle the garlic powder evenly over the slices. Bake until the garlic bread is golden brown and toasted, about 20 minutes (but keep an eye on it). Serve warm.

Tata's Cuban Rice with Secret Sofrito _____

Serves 4

This classic Cuban dish is simple, filling, nutritious, and ultimately kid-friendly because of its mild, appealing flavors and textures. It also contains *sofrito*, a kind of core base of sautéed vegetables for a sauce. Many different cultures have their own signature combinations. Cuban *sofrito* is a bit different than Italian or Spanish *sofrito*—it is characterized by garlic, sweet peppers, and onions, with or without tomatoes, and sautéed with herbs and spices, typically bay leaves, cumin, and oregano. Each of these seasonings contains many beneficial and healing phytochemicals, and the black beans add protein (although you can also make this as a side dish without the beans).

I like to make *sofrito* the way Tata did—a simple version with a flavor that appeals to children. Cooking the *sofrito* thoroughly before adding it to simple foods such as rice or pasta sauce allows the vegetables practically to melt away, making them delicious but indistinguishable—no icky vegetable "pieces" that offend some children.

> 1 cup enriched long-grain white rice or basmati brown rice
> 2 1/2 cups organic vegetable broth for cooking the rice, plus an
>   additional 1/4 cup
> 1 tablespoon olive oil
> 4 garlic cloves, peeled and minced
> 1 large onion (white or yellow), peeled and chopped finely
> 1 large green bell pepper, or 2 cubanelle peppers, cored and minced
> 1 teaspoon salt
> 1 (15-ounce) can organic black beans, drained and rinsed

> *Optional garnish:*
> 1 tablespoon minced fresh cilantro

Prepare the rice according to the package directions, using 2 to 2 1/2 cups of organic vegetable broth instead of water. While the rice is cooking, heat the olive oil in a large skillet over medium heat. Add the garlic, onion, peppers, and salt. Cook slowly, stirring frequently to avoid browning, until the vegetables are very soft and begin to combine, about 20 minutes. Add the remaining 1/4 cup of vegetable broth and simmer until the vegetables begin to dissolve.

When the rice is tender, stir in the vegetable mixture and the beans. Serve warm.

Bean Burritos

Serves 4

These yummy, protein-rich, fiber-full, vitamin-packed burritos are kid-friendly and easy to pick up and eat. Serve with salsa and/or guacamole for dipping or topping.

Cooking spray
1 cup organic vegetarian refried beans
1/2 cup cooked long-grain brown rice
1/2 cup grated fresh organic cauliflower (use a regular box grater
    and grate it like cheese)
1/2 cup vegetable broth
1/2 teaspoon salt
4 (6-inch) whole-grain organic tortillas
1/2 cup shredded vegan cheese (or organic cheddar, if you are
    transitioning)

Preheat the oven to 375°F. Spray a 13 by 9-inch baking pan with cooking spray.

In a large saucepan, combine the refried beans, cooked rice, grated cauliflower, vegetable broth, and salt. Heat over medium heat, stirring occasionally, until hot and bubbly.

Heat a tortilla in a dry skillet over medium heat just until soft. Put it in the baking pan. Top with one-quarter of the bean mixture and one-quarter of the cheese. Turn the ends over, and then roll up the tortilla tightly. Repeat with the remaining tortillas.

Bake until the tortillas are firm and crispy, about 40 minutes. Serve with your favorite toppings.

Grilled PB&J

Serves 1. Can be doubled, tripled, or more.

Sweet, gooey, warm, and melty—it's lunch and dessert all in one! When you use whole-grain bread, this meal has plenty of fiber. Sourdough bread has been shown to stabilize blood sugar levels even better than other kinds of bread. Either way, your children win.

   2 slices whole-grain or sourdough bread
   1 tablespoon natural peanut butter
   1 tablespoon all-fruit jam (or leftover strawberry sauce from
        pancakes, page 230)
   2 teaspoons trans-fat-free nondairy butter (e.g., Earth Balance)

Heat a skillet over medium heat. Spread one slice of bread with peanut butter. Spread the other slice with jam. Put the peanut butter–jam sides together to make a sandwich. Spread 1 teaspoon of butter on each outer surface of the sandwich. Put the sandwich in the skillet and fry until golden and crispy. Flip over and cook the other side. Transfer to a plate. Cut the sandwich into four triangles. Serve warm.

Peanut Butter Roll-Ups

Serves 1. Can be doubled, tripled, or more.

Peanut butter is protein-rich and filling, so your child will stay satisfied and have level energy for hours afterward.

   1 whole-grain tortilla
   1 tablespoon peanut butter

   Optional toppings:
   1 tablespoon all-fruit spread
   1 banana, sliced
   1 tablespoon chopped pecans
   1 tablespoon real maple syrup
   Mini vegan chocolate chips (a tiny bit of sugar is okay every so
        often for kids who aren't sugar sensitive)

Warm the tortilla in a dry skillet over medium heat just until it softens. Put the tortilla on a plate and spread with the peanut butter. Add your choice of additional toppings evenly over the peanut butter. Roll the tortilla tightly and serve, or slice into bite-size disks and serve.

Sweet Snacks and Desserts

Magic Mix

Serves any number

This fun and easy trail mix is as magical and unique as your children. You supply the possible ingredients, your children choose their own individual combinations, and it's snacktime. This mix is healthy and filling. No more between-meal munchies!

Suggested toppings:
Peanuts
Almonds
Walnuts
Raisins
Dried cranberries
Dried cherries
Dried blueberries
Vegan chocolate chips
Coconut flakes
Banana chips
Dried apple rings
Mini organic pretzels
Favorite whole-grain cereal, such as crisp rice, oat O's, peanut
    butter puffs, corn squares, and so on (look for naturally
    sweetened)

Put out bowls of toppings. Each child gets his or her own resealable bag. Instruct the children to fill each bag halfway, so there is room for shaking. (Each bag should contain no more than 1 tablespoon of chocolate chips.) Shake up the mixture and enjoy.

Nicki's Almond Nut Butter Boats _____

Serves 1 or 2, depending on hunger

My daughter, Nicki, made up this fanciful treat. It contains almond butter, a luscious alternative to peanut butter, full of healthy nut oil, plus calcium, iron, and zinc.

1 banana
1 tablespoon any nut butter
1 tablespoon raisins

This is Nicki's original recipe.

Peel the banana. Slice out an opening along the top like a boat. Fill with the nut butter and top with raisins (the passengers). For serving or presentation, use four toothpicks inserted along the bottom sides at a diagonal, to make the boat stand upright. Serve as a fun finger food—and remove the toothpicks before handing to a small child!

Cinnamon Cream _____

Serves 2. Can be doubled.

Even nondairy yogurts are typically fortified with calcium, some have added fiber, and cinnamon minimizes blood sugar crashes.

6 to 8 ounces coconut, soy, or dairy yogurt, plain or vanilla-flavored
1 tablespoon real maple syrup, if the yogurt is plain
1/4 teaspoon ground cinnamon

Combine all the ingredients and keep chilled. Use for dipping fruit chunks or making fruit parfaits.

Nanny Fruit _____

Just fill individual bowls with fruit cut into bite-size pieces and sprinkle with a pinch of ground cinnamon, a spoonful of shredded coconut, a sprinkle of sliced almonds, and a drizzle of real maple syrup. Delicious!

L.O.V.E. Cupcakes

Makes 12 cupcakes

These sweet and delicate cupcakes with a light, fluffy chocolate frosting are sweetened entirely with agave syrup, not sugar, and made with whole-grain flour, not white flour. The soy milk and powder provide healthful protein without the addition of dairy products. Try to use as many organic products in these cupcakes as you can. In the ingredient list, I've listed a few brands I like.

This recipe is based on Simple Vanilla and Agave Nectar Cupcakes from *Vegan Cupcakes Take Over the World*, by Isa Chandra Moskowitz and Terry Hope Romero, a wonderful collection of dairy-free cupcakes. I love how sweet and festive these cupcakes are, especially when you pipe on the icing and top each cupcake with a strawberry or raspberry. L.O.V.E. without guilt!

2/3 cup organic soy milk
1/2 teaspoon Bragg organic, raw, unfiltered apple cider vinegar
2/3 cup organic light agave nectar (I like Madhava brand)
1/3 cup canola oil
1 1/2 teaspoons vanilla extract
1/2 teaspoon almond extract
1 1/3 cups organic whole wheat pastry flour or white whole wheat
    flour (whichever you have)
3/4 teaspoon baking powder
1/2 teaspoon baking soda
1/4 teaspoon sea salt

Frosting:
1/2 cup (1 stick) Earth Balance margarine, softened to room
    temperature
1/2 cup organic light agave syrup
1 1/2 teaspoons vanilla extract
1/2 cup organic unsweetened cocoa powder, sifted (I use Equal
    Exchange organic and fairly traded baking cocoa)
1/2 cup plain soy milk powder (find this in the natural foods section
    of your grocery store or in the bulk bins at your natural foods
    market—it's just pure roasted soybeans ground to a powder)

Optional:
12 small strawberries or raspberries, for garnish

Make the cupcakes:
Preheat the oven to 325°F. In a large bowl, combine the soy milk and vinegar. Let it sit for 5 minutes, to curdle the soy milk (this adds a buttermilk-like flavor). Put paper liners in a twelve-cup muffin pan.

Add the agave syrup, oil, and vanilla and almond extract to the soy milk mixture and beat with a fork until completely combined. Sift in the flour, baking powder, baking soda, and salt. Mix with a fork or electric beater on low until smooth. Pour the batter into the prepared pan, filling the cups no more than three-quarters full.

Bake for 20 minutes, or until a toothpick inserted into the center of a cupcake comes out clean. Do not overbake these cupcakes, or they will be dry.

Cool the cupcakes completely on a wire rack, at least for 1 hour. The texture and flavor gets better as the cupcakes cool, and they need to be completely cool before frosting.

As the cupcakes cool, make the frosting:
In a large bowl, combine the margarine and agave syrup. Beat with an electric mixer until smooth. Whisk in the vanilla, then slowly fold in the cocoa powder so it doesn't poof all over your counter.

When the cocoa powder is mostly coated with margarine, beat it with an electric mixer on medium speed until the frosting begins to get fluffy. Add the soy milk powder, one spoonful at a time, and continue to beat on low speed until all of it is incorporated. If the frosting seems too soft, add a little more soy milk powder. If it seems too stiff, add a little more agave syrup.

Frost the cooled cupcakes with a knife, or pipe it on with a pastry bag and star tip. Optional: Top each cupcake with a fresh berry.

Appendix Two

Organic Nanny Resources

There are so many wonderful resources out there that can help mamas and papas live a more natural, organic life. Here are just a few of my favorites. Let them inspire you to seek out even more information. The more you know, the easier it will be to live with L.O.V.E.

Web Sites

Animal Welfare
ASPCA: www.aspca.org
Farm Sanctuary: www.farmsanctuary.com
Humane Society: www.humanesociety.org
PETA: www.peta.org

Attachment Parenting
Attachment Parenting International: www.attachmentparenting.org/pdfs/API
    _Safe_Infant_Sleep_brochure.pdf
Ask Dr. Sears: www.askdrsears.com

Community-Supported Agriculture
Biodynamic Farming and Gardening Association: www.biodynamics.com/csa1
    .html
Local Harvest: www.localharvest.org
National Sustainable Agriculture Information Service: http://attra.ncat.org
    /attra-pub.local_food

Consumer Safety
Air Purifiers: www.air-purifiers-america.com
Campaign for Safe Cosmetics: www.safecosmetics.org
Environmental Working Group: www.ewg.org

Co-Ops

Co-op Directory Service: www.coopdirectory.org/directory.htm
Cooperative Grocer: www.cooperativegrocer.coop/coops
Local Harvest: www.localharvest.org

Farmers' Markets

FarmersMarket.com: www.farmersmarket.com
Farmer's Market Online: www.farmersmarketonline.com/Openair.htm

Gluten-Free

Celiac Chicks: www.celiacchicks.com
Celiac Disease Foundation: www.celiac.org
Celiac.com: www.celiac.com/catalog/product_info.php?products_id=467
The Gluten Free Casein Free Diet: www.gfcfdiet.com

Natural Food Home Delivery

Diamond Organics: www.diamondorganics.com
Frontier Natural Brands: www.frontiercoop.com
Gold Mine Natural Foods: www.goldminenaturalfoods.com
Jaffe Bros. Natural Foods: www.organicfruitsandnuts.com

Vegan, Vegetarian, and Raw Restaurants

Happy Cow: www.happycow.net
Veg Dining: www.vegdining.com/Home.cfm
Vegetarian-Restaurants.net: www.vegetarian-restaurants.net/usa/index.html
All Raw Directory: www.allrawdirectory.com/rawfoods.asp?topic=rawfood
    restaurants

Vegan/Vegetarian Information

Choose Veg: http://chooseveg.com
PCRM: www.pcrm.org
T. Colin Campbell: www.tcolincampbell.org
The Vegetarian Resource Group: www.vrg.org
Vegan MD: http://veganmd.com

Water

Clean Water Action: www.cleanwateraction.org/Guide to Tap Water Filtration
Food and Water Watch: www.foodandwaterwatch.org/take-action/consumer-tools
    /choosing-a-water-filter
WellOwner.org: www.wellowner.org

Music

The Happiest Baby on the Block: New "Super Soothing" Calming Sounds by Harvey
    Karp, MD
Lullabies for Sleepy Eyes by Susie Tallman

More from Pooh Corner by Kenny Loggins
Quiet Time by Raffi
Return to Pooh Corner by Kenny Loggins
Traditional Lullabies by Growing Minds with Music

Cookbooks

1,000 Vegan Recipes by Robin Robertson
Ani's Raw Food Essentials: Recipes and Techniques for Mastering the Art of Raw Food by Ani Phyo
Better Than Peanut Butter & Jelly: Quick Vegetarian Meals Your Kids Will Love! by Marty Mattare and Wendy Muldawer
The Candle Café Cookbook: More than 150 Recipes from New York's Renowned Vegan Restaurant by Joy Pierson, Bart Protenza, and Barbara Scott-Goodman
The Complete Guide to Vegan Food Substitutions: Veganize It! Foolproof Methods for Transforming Any Dish into a Delicious New Vegan Favorite by Celine Steen and Joni Marie Newman
The Conscious Cook: Delicious Meatless Meals That Will Change the Way You Eat by Tal Ronnen
The Gluten-Free Vegan: 150 Delicious Gluten-Free, Animal-Free Recipes by Susan O'Brien
Happy, Healthy, Vegan Kids: With Vegan and Gluten-Free Recipes by Tracie DeMotte
The Happy Herbivore: Over 175 Delicious Fat-Free and Low-Fat Vegan Recipes by Lindsay S. Nixon
The Real Food Daily Cookbook: Really Fresh, Really Good, Really Vegetarian by Ann Gentry and Anthony Head
The Ultimate Uncheese Cookbook: Delicious Dairy-Free Cheeses and Classic "Uncheese" Dishes by Jo Stepaniak
Vegan Cupcakes Take Over the World: 75 Dairy-Free Recipes for Cupcakes That Rule by Isa Chandra Moskowitz and Terry Hope Romero
Vegan Lunch Box: 130 Amazing, Animal-Free Lunches Kids and Grown-Ups Will Love! by Jennifer McCann
The Vegan Table: 200 Unforgettable Recipes for Entertaining Every Guest at Every Occasion by Colleen Patrick-Goudreau
Veganomicon: The Ultimate Vegan Cookbook by Isa Chandra Moskowitz and Terry Hope Romero
Vegan's Daily Companion: 365 Days of Inspiration for Cooking, Eating, and Living Compassionately by Colleen Patrick-Goudreau
Viva Vegan!: 200 Authentic and Fabulous Recipes for Latin Food Lovers by Terry Hope Romero
Vive le Vegan!: Simple Delectable Recipes for the Everyday Vegan Family by Dreena Burton

Children's Books

Children Make Terrible Pets by Peter Brown

Emma and Mommy Talk to God by Marianne Williamson
Herb the Vegetarian Dragon by Jules Bass
Hubert the Pudge: A Vegetarian Tale by Henrik Drescher
I Think, I Am!: Teaching Kids the Power of Affirmations by Louise L. Hay
Interrupting Chicken by David Ezra Stein
Mary Poppins by P. L. Travers
No Excuses!: How What You Say Can Get in Your Way by Wayne W. Dyer
On My Way to a Happy Life by Deepak Chopra
A Pig Parade Is a Terrible Idea by Michael Ian Black
A Sick Day for Amos McGee by Philip Christian Stead
The Tale of Peter Rabbit by Beatrix Potter
That's Why We Don't Eat Animals by Ruby Roth
Unstoppable Me!: 10 Ways to Soar Through Life by Wayne W. Dyer

Reading List for Mamas

Attached at the Heart: 8 Proven Parenting Principles for Raising Connected and Compassionate Children by Barbara Nicholson and Lysa Parker
The Attachment Parenting Book by Williams Sears, MD, and Martha Sears, RN
The China Study by Colin T. Campbell, PhD, and Thomas M. Campbell II
The Complete Idiot's Guide to Gluten-Free Eating by Eve Adamson
Crazy Sexy Diet: Eat Your Veggies, Ignite Your Spark, and Live Like You Mean It! by Kris Carr
Diet for a New America by John Robbins
Disease-Proof Your Child: Feeding Kids Right by Joel Fuhrman, MD
Dr. Spock's Baby & Child by Benjamin Spock, MD
Eating Animals by Jonathan Safran Foer
Food Rules: An Eater's Manual by Michael Pollan
Gorgeously Green: 8 Simple Steps to an Earth-Friendly Life by Sophie Uliano
The Green Book by Elizabeth Rogers
Healthy Child, Healthy World: Creating a Cleaner, Greener, Safer Home by Christopher Gavigan
How to Talk So Kids Will Listen & Listen So Kids Will Talk by Adele Faber and Elaine Mazlish
Pets Gone Green: Live a More Eco-Conscious Life with Your Pets by Eve Adamson
Raising Vegan Children in a Non-Vegan World: A Complete Guide for Parents by Erin Pavlina
Raising Vegetarian Children: A Guide to Good Health and Family Harmony by Joanne Stepaniak and Vesanto Melina
The Secret by Rhonda Byrnes
Skinny Bitch by Rory Freedman and Kim Barnouin
You Can Heal Your Life by Louise L. Hay
You'll See It When You Believe It by Dr. Wayne Dyer

Index

Addiction
  cheese, 78
  junk food, 15–16, 53, 128, 152–153
  sugar, 52–53, 55
  white flour, 68
  ADHD (attention
    deficithyperactivity disorder), 30,
    55, 56, 135
Affirmation meditation, 160
Albom, Mitch, 198
Almond Nut Butter Boats, Nicki's, 244
American Celiac Disease Alliance, 73
American Dietetic Association,
    100–101
American Heart Association, 13, 15
Angelou, Maya, 147
Animal products. *See* Meat
    consumption; Vegetable-centric,
    vegetarian, or vegan lifestyle
Animal rights organizations, 196
Animals, compassion for, 102, 195–196
Annals of Nutrition and Metabolism, 34
Archives of Internal Medicine, 99
Artificial ingredients, 32, 35–37
Aspartame, 36
  Attention deficithyperactivity
    disorder (ADHD), 30, 55, 56, 135
Autism, 73, 81, 135, 179
Avon Longitudinal Study of Parents
    and Children, 29

Back-to-Basics Smoothie, 227–228
Barnard, Neal, 78

Baths
  herbs and essential oils for, 174, 177
  as natural remedy, 174, 177
  purity of bath products, 141–143
  scrubs and spa treatments, 157–159
Beans
  Bean Burritos, 241
  Hummus, 233–234
  Tata's Cuban Rice with Secret
    Sofrito, 240–241
Behavioral problems
  diet and, 12–14, 30
  discipline for, 215–220
  sugar and, 20, 51–52, 54–55, 56–58
  trans fats and, 33
Beverages
  Back-to-Basics Smoothie, 227–228
  diet upgrade, 124–125
  Orange-Strawberry Smoothie, 229
  Organic Nanny Juice, 225–226
  Organic Nanny Smoothie, 227–228
  Purple Power Smoothie, 228
  Secret Agent Smoothie, 228–229
  smoothie for mothers, 156
  Tata's Smooth Move Juice Remedy,
    180
  teas, 181
  water, 41, 151, 182
  wheatgrass, 156, 162
Birmingham, Carolyn, 220
Blueberry Pancakes with Strawberry
    Sauce, 229–231
Bogalusa Heart Study, 13

Brain development and IQ, 29–30, 92, 135
Breakfast foods. *See also* Smoothies
　Blueberry Pancakes with Strawberry Sauce, 229–231
　Fried Tofu Breakfast Sandwich, 231
　L.O.V.E. Muffins, 232
　menus, 118–119, 154
　protein in, 54, 125
Breastfeeding, 116
Burke, Leo J., 173
Burritos, Bean, 241
Bush, George H. W., 109

Calcium, 81, 105. *See also* Dairy products
Calendula Skin Cream, Tata's Cuban, 190
Campaign for Safe Cosmetics (CSC), 143
Campbell, T. Colin, 77
Cancer risk
　chemical exposure, 134, 143
　dairy consumption, 77
　meat consumption, 99
　processed-meat consumption, 36
Canfield, Jack, 221
Carson, Rachel, 135
Castor oil massage, 181
Celiac disease, 73
Centers for Disease Control and Prevention, 73
Cheese. *See also* Dairy products
　addictiveness, 78
　dairy-free, 82
　flavor alternative, 105, 127
Chemicals
　artificial food additives, 32, 35–37
　cleaning products, 139–141
　personal hygiene products, 141–143
　pesticides, 92, 94, 134, 137
　risks to children, 134–135
　volatile organic compounds, 136–138

Child, Julia, 27
Childhood obesity
　fast food, 29
　heart disease risk, 13–14
　high-fructose corn syrup, 34–35
　rate of, 15, 34
　white flour, 65–67, 68
Cinnamon Cream, 244
Clean 15 and Dirty Dozen foods, 94–95
Cleaner, Organic Nanny, 140
Cleaning products, 139–141
Cleansing, internal
　constipation remedies, 69, 179–181
　hydration, 181–182
　raw-food cleanse, 155–157
Colds and coughs, 181, 188–189
Community Supported Agriculture (CSA), 91
Composting, 204
Constipation, 69, 179–181
Convenience food. *See* De-junking children; Fast food and junk food
Cooking from scratch, 19, 117–122
Co-sleeping, 186–188
Cough Syrup, Organic Nanny, 189
Cox, Marcelene, 11
Cream, Cinnamon, 244
CSA (Community Supported Agriculture), 91
CSC (Campaign for Safe Cosmetics), 143
Cuban Mashed Sweet Potatoes, 235–236
Cuban Rice with Secret Sofrito, Tata's, 240–241
Cuban Salsa, 234
Cuban Sugar Scrub, 158
Cupcakes, L.O.V.E., 245–246

Dairy products
　addictiveness of cheese, 78
　calcium-rich alternatives, 81

cheese-flavor alternative, 105, 127
industrial milk production, 83
organic, 93
phasing out, 21, 81–83
problems associated with, 75–81
to-do list, 84
De-junking children. *See also* L.O.V.E.,
    transition to
artificial ingredients, 32, 35–37
assessment of current patterns, 22
changing habits, 17–19, 25, 30, 32
DIY Happier Meals, 48
fast food, 42–48
good snacks, 39
as gradual process, 20, 23, 25
high-fructose corn syrup, 32,
    34–35
importance of, 29–30
quality spectrum of processed
    foods, 40–41
single worst item, 28, 30–32
three-step approach, 37–42
trans fats, 32–34
water consumption, 41
to-do lists, 26, 49
Depressive behavior
sugar and, 20, 54, 57
trans fats and, 33
Desserts. *See* Sweet snacks and
    desserts
Detoxing children. *See* De-junking
    children
Detoxing home. *See* Home
    environment
Dietary fiber, 69
Digestive problems, 69, 179–181
Dips
    Cuban Salsa, 234
    Hummus, 233–234
    Simple Guacamole, 233
Dirty Dozen and Clean 15 foods,
    94–95
Discipline, 215–220
DIY Happier Meals, 48

Doctors, holistic, 175
Drinks. *See* Beverages
Dyer, Wayne, 197

Emotional eating, 152–153, 212–213
Energy loss
    energy foods, 166
    energy tips, 162
    exercise and, 161–166
    from poor diet, 12
Environment, indoor. *See* Home
    environment
Environmental consciousness
    easy actions, 107–108, 143–145
    groundwater pollution, 139
    in L.O.V.E. principles, 106–107
    time spent outdoors, 196–197
Environmental Working Group,
    94–95, 143
Essential oils
    in cleaning products, 141
    for therapy, 165, 177–178, 188
Exercise, 161–166

Family Circle, 54
Fast food and junk food. *See also*
    De-junking children
    addictiveness, 15–16, 53, 128,
    152–153
    enticement of children,
    "McDonald's Effect," 43, 99
    problems associated with, 13–15,
    29–30
    SAD (standard American diet),
    12–13, 16–17
    science experiment with, 47
Fiber, dietary, 69
Flour, eliminating from diet, 70, 72. *See
    also* White flour
Food, Inc. (movie), 44
Framingham Children's Study, 14
French Fries, Homemade, 234–235
Fried Tofu Breakfast Sandwich, 231
Fruit, Nanny, 244

Fruits and vegetables, pesticide
    residue in, 92, 94–95

Gardening, 203–206
Garlic Bread, Whole-Grain, 239
Global Volunteers, 200
Gluten Free Casein Free Diet (GFCF),
    73
Gluten sensitivity, 73, 81
Gratitude
    compassion for animals, 102,
        195–196
    daily thanksgiving, 201–203
    exposure to natural world, 196–197
    gardening, 203–206
    journaling, 201
    reinforcement of selflessness and
        empathy, 205
    saying "thank you," 202
    service to others, 197–201
    vision boards, 206–207
    to-do list, 207
Green Salad, 236
Grilled PB&J, 242
Guacamole, Simple, 233

Happier Meals, DIY, 48
Happy Meals, McDonald's, 46
Harvard University, 53, 99
H.E.A.L. mealtime strategies, 110
Healing. *See* Natural remedies
Healthy Child, Healthy World
    organization, 134
Heart disease risk
    childhood obesity, 13–14
    meat consumption, 99
    trans fat consumption, 34
    vegetarian diet and, 101
Hemp fabric, 138
Herbs and essential oils
    baths, 177–178
    cleaning products, 141
    for colds and coughs, 181, 188–189
    massage oil, 165

skin cream, 190
teas, 181
High-fructose corn syrup (HFCS),
    34–35
Holistic doctors, 175
Home environment
    cleaning products, 139–141
    indoor air pollution, 136–138
    personal hygiene products, 141–143
    toxins in, 133–135
    to-do list, 146
Homemade French Fries, 234–235
Homemade Happier Meals, 48
Hummus, 233–234
Hydration, 41, 151, 181–182
Hyman, Mark, 53
Hyperactivity, 20, 30, 54–55, 56

Illness. *See* Natural remedies
Intuitive parenting
    discipline, 215–220
    listening to child, 211–215
    parent's time-out, 216, 218
    trust in intuition, 209–211, 221–223
    to-do list, 223
IQ, 29–30, 92, 135

Jensen, Bernard, 133
Journals, 201
Juices. *See also* Smoothies
    diet upgrade, 124–125
    Organic Nanny Juice, 225–226
    Tata's Smooth Move Juice Remedy,
        180
    wheatgrass, 156, 162
Junk food. *See* De-junking children;
        Fast food and junk food

Kay, John, 145
Kozol, Jonathan, 114
Kradjian, Robert M., 80

Listening to child, 211–215
Local food and lifestyle, 88–90, 91

Local Harvest, 91
London, William, 176
Lourie, Bruce, *Slow Death by Rubber Duck*, 141
L.O.V.E. Cupcakes, 245–246
L.O.V.E. Muffins, 232
L.O.V.E. principles
  environmental awareness, 106–108
  as guide to well-being, 23–25, 87–88
  local food and lifestyle, 88–90, 91
  organic food and lifestyle, 90–96
  vegetable-centric, vegetarian, or vegan lifestyle, 96–106
  to-do list, 108
L.O.V.E., transition to. *See also* Dejunking children
  for babies, 112–115
  cooking from scratch, 19, 117–122
  H.E.A.L. strategies, 110
  health improvements, 130
  juices and smoothies, 124–125
  mealtime ideas, 129–131
  menu, 116–119
  parental authority and leadership, 131–132
  for picky eaters, 111–112, 122
  relaxed mealtime, 121
  snacks, 126–128
  stealth health, 122–124
  for toddlers, 115–116
  to-do list, 132

Magic Mix, 243
Main dishes
  Bean Burritos, 241
  Grilled PB&J, 242
  Make-Your-Own Pizzas, 238
  Organic Nanny Tacos, 236–237
  Pasta with Red Sauce, 238–239
  Peanut Butter Roll-Ups, 242–243
  Tata's Cuban Rice with Secret Sofrito, 240–241
  Tofu Fingers, 237
Make-Your-Own Pizzas, 238

Manning, Anita, 95
Mashed Potatoes, Organic Nanny, 235
Mashed Sweet Potatoes, Cuban, 235–236
Massage, 165, 181, 184
Massage Oil, Organic Nanny, 158
"McDonald's Effect," 43, 99
McDonald's Happy Meals, 47
Meat consumption
  as emotional issue, 101–102
  health problems associated with, 99–100
  industrial meat production, 97, 106–107
  lifetime eating habits, 99–101
  organic meat, 93–94, 103
  phasing out, 21, 97, 103–104
  for special occasions, 96–97
  in United States, 96
  upgrading, 97, 103
Meditation, 159–161
Menus
  for children, 116–119
  for mothers, 154
Meyer, Paul J., 167
Milk. *See* Dairy products
"Milk Letter," 80
Monosodium glutamate (MSG), 36, 128
Montessori, Maria, 218
Mother Teresa, 218
Mothering. *See* Intuitive parenting
Mothers
  exercise, 161–166
  female friendships, 168–169
  help with emotional healing, 153
  L.O.V.E. foods, 150–155
  makeover changes, 149–150
  massage, 165
  morning meditation, 159–161
  sleep, 164, 185–186
  snacks, 156
  spa Sundays, 155–159
  spirituality, 166–168

Mothers (*continued*)
    stress and self-neglect, 147–149
    teaching children by example, 30,
        131, 169–171
    to-do list, 170
MSG (monosodium glutamate), 128,
    141–143
Muffins, L.O.V.E., 232

Nanny Fruit, 244
National Sleep Foundation, 183
Natural remedies
    baths, 174, 177–179
    calmness, 176
    for colds and coughs, 181,
        188–189
    for constipation, 69, 179–181
    five-step approach to healing, 176
    fresh air and sunshine, 191
    herbs and essential oils, 177–179,
        181, 188
    hydration, 41, 181–182
    L.O.V.E. foods, 191
    rest, 182–188
    for skin irritation and dryness,
        189–191
    teas, 181
    when to call doctor, 175
    to-do list, 192
Nicki's Almond Nut Butter Boats, 244
Nitrates and nitrites, 36
Nutritional yeast, 105, 127

Obesity
    fast food, 29
    heart disease risk, 13–14
    high-fructose corn syrup, 34–35
    rate of, 15, 34
    white flour, 65–67, 68
Orange-Strawberry Smoothie, 229
Organic life
    bath products, 141–143
    cleaning products, 139–141
    cost of organic food, 92–93, 203

    environmental benefits, 107
    gardening, 203–206
    indoor air quality, 136–138
    meats and dairy products, 93–94,
        103
    phasing in, 94–96
    purity and safety, 90–94
Organic Nanny Cough Syrup, 189
Organic Nanny Juice, 225–226
Organic Nanny Mashed Potatoes,
    235
Organic Nanny Massage Oil, 158
Organic Nanny Smoothie, 227–228
Organic Nanny Tacos, 236–237

Pancakes, Blueberry, with Strawberry
    Sauce, 229–231
Parent self-care. *See* Mothers
Parenting. *See* Intuitive parenting
Pasta with Red Sauce, 238–239
Peanut butter
    Grilled PB&J, 242
    Peanut Butter Roll-Ups, 242–243
Pediatrics, 29
Personal care products
    Cuban Sugar Scrub, 158
    nontoxic bath products, 141–143
    Organic Nanny Massage Oil, 158
    Sea Salt Scrub, 158
    spa treatments, 157–159
    Tata's Cuban Calendula Skin
        Cream, 190
Pesticides, 92, 94–95, 134, 137
*Pharmacology, Biochemistry and
    Behavior*, 34–35
Pizzas, Make-Your-Own, 238
Plant-based diet, 99, 130, 150–151. *See
    also* Vegetable-centric,
    vegetarian, or vegan lifestyle
Pollan, Michael, 11
Potatoes
    Homemade French Fries, 234–235
    Organic Nanny Mashed Potatoes,
        235

Processed food. *See* De-junking
  children; Fast food and junk food;
  Sugar; White flour
Produce, pesticide residue in, 92,
  94–95
Protein foods
  addition to smoothies, 125
  reduction of sugar craving, 52, 54
  in vegetarian diet, 102, 105
Purees for stealth health, 122–124
Purple Power Smoothie, 228

Ram, Bhava, 206
Raw-food cleanse, 155–157
Red Sauce, Pasta with, 238–239
Rewards for good behavior, 218–219
Rice with Secret Sofrito, Tata's Cuban,
  240–241
Roll-Ups, Peanut Butter, 242–243
Roth, Ruby, *That's Why We Don't Eat
  Animals*, 100

SAD (standard American diet), 12–13,
  16–17
Salad, Green, 236
Salsa, Cuban, 234
Sandwiches
  Fried Tofu Breakfast Sandwich,
    231
  Grilled PB&J, 242
  Peanut Butter Roll-Ups, 242–243
Scripps Research Institute, 16
Scrubs and spa treatments, 157–159
Secret ingredients
  juices and smoothies, 124–125
  Pasta with Red Sauce, 238–239
  purees, 122–124
  Secret Agent Smoothie, 228–229
  Tata's Cuban Rice with Secret
    Sofrito, 240–241
Self-care for mothers. *See* Mothers
Service to others, 197–201
Shaw, George Bernard, 85
Sickness. *See* Natural remedies

Side dishes
  Cuban Mashed Sweet Potatoes,
    235–236
  Green Salad, 236
  Homemade French Fries, 234–235
  Organic Nanny Mashed Potatoes,
    235
  Whole-Grain Garlic Bread, 239
Sierra Club, 200
Simple Guacamole, 233
Skin Cream, Tata's Cuban Calendula,
  190
Skin irritation and dryness, 189–191
Sleep
  bedtime strategies, 183–186
  co-sleeping, 186–188
  for mothers, 164, 185–186
  as natural remedy, 182–188
  requirements, 183
Sleepytime Tray, 184
Slow Death by Rubber Duck (Smith and
  Lourie), 141
Smoothies
  Back-to-Basics Smoothie, 227–228
  for children, 124–125
  for mothers, 156
  Orange-Strawberry Smoothie, 229
  Organic Nanny Smoothie, 227–228
  Purple Power Smoothie, 228
  Secret Agent Smoothie, 228–229
Snacks. *See also* Dips; Sweet snacks
    and desserts
  at bedtime, 184
  menus, 118–119, 154
  for mothers, 156
  sweet treats, 62–63
  for travel, 39
  for upgrading diet, 39, 126–128
Sofrito, Tata's Cuban Rice with Secret,
  240–241
Spa Sundays, 155–159
Spirituality, 166–168
Spock, Benjamin, 76, 109, 209
Sprouted-grain bread, 71

Stealth health
    juices and smoothies, 124–125
    Pasta with Red Sauce, 238–239
    purees, 122–124
    Secret Agent Smoothie, 228–229
    Tata's Cuban Rice with Secret
        Sofrito, 240–241
Strawberries
    Blueberry Pancakes with
        Strawberry Sauce, 229–231
    Orange-Strawberry Smoothie, 229
Sugar
    addictiveness, 52–53, 55
    alternatives, 61–63
    behavioral problems associated
        with, 20, 51–52, 54–55, 56–58
    as body scrub, 57, 158
    effect on blood sugar, 20, 55, 56
    versus high-fructose corn syrup,
        34–35
    immune system response, 54–55
    phasing out, 20, 59–64
    replacement with protein, 52, 54
    symptoms of sugar sensitivity,
        56–58
    to-do list, 63
Sugar-Free Toddlers (Watson), 55
Super Size Me (movie), 43, 44
Sweet Potatoes, Cuban Mashed,
    235–236
Sweet snacks and desserts
    Cinnamon Cream, 244
    L.O.V.E. Cupcakes, 245–246
    Magic Mix, 243
    Nanny Fruit, 244
    Nicki's Almond Nut Butter Boats,
        244
    sweet additions to smoothies,
        125
    sweet treats, 62–63
Swindoll, Charles, 222

Tacos, Organic Nanny, 236–237
Tantrums, 217

Tata's Cuban Calendula Skin Cream,
    190
Tata's Cuban Rice with Secret Sofrito,
    240–241
Tata's Smooth Move Juice Remedy,
    180
Teas, 181
Thankfulness. *See* Gratitude
That's Why We Don't Eat Animals
    (Roth), 100
Therapy-dog certification, 200–201
Tillich, Paul, 214
Time magazine, 106
Time-outs, 217
Tofu
    Fried Tofu Breakfast Sandwich,
        231
    Tofu Fingers, 237
Toxins. *See* Chemicals
Trail mix, 243
Trans fats, 32–34
Treats. *See* Sweet snacks and desserts

University of California at Davis, 201
University of California at Los
    Angeles, 169
University of Michigan, 166–167
University of North Carolina, 13–14
Upgrading diet. *See* L.O.V.E., transition
    to
U.S. Food and Drug Administration,
    192

Validation of child's feelings, 212–214,
    219
Vegetable-centric, vegetarian, or
    vegan lifestyle
    American Dietetic Association on,
        100–101
    farm field trip, 102
    health benefits, 99–100
    inspiration and encouragement for,
        97, 100
    Meatless Monday, 103

nutritional concerns, 101, 102, 105, 162

personal products and clothes, 105–106

phasing in, 103–105

terms describing, 98

well-being of vegan family, 85–86

Vegetables and fruits, pesticide residue in, 92, 94–95

Vision boards, 167–168, 206–207

Vitamin B$_{12}$, 101, 105, 162

Volatile organic compounds (VOC), 136–138

Volunteer opportunities, 197–201

Water consumption, 41, 151, 182

Watson, Susan, *Sugar-Free Toddlers*, 55

Wheat, 67–68, 73. *See also* White flour

Wheatgrass, 156, 162

White flour
  addictiveness, 68
  effect on blood sugar, 68–69
  lack of fiber, 69

obesity and, 65–67

phasing out, 21, 70–72

symptoms of excessive consumption, 69–70

wheat, 67–68, 73

Whole foods. *See also* L.O.V.E., transition to
  as convenient option, 18–19
  effect on health and behavior, 14–15, 130, 150–151
  sugar cane and natural sweeteners, 58–59, 61

Whole grains
  fiber in, 69
  phasing in, 70–72
  sprouted-grain bread, 71
  in whole form, 70, 72
  to-do list, 74

Whole-Grain Garlic Bread, 239

Wigmore, Ann, 148

Willett, Walter C., 76

Winfrey, Oprah, 193

World Health Organization, 73, 99

Worldwatch Institute, 106